DISCOVER
COLOR THERAPY

DISCOVER
COLOR THERAPY

HELEN GRAHAM

KATHERINE ARMITAGE
Illustrator

Ulysses Press 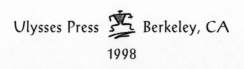 Berkeley, CA
1998

This book has been written and published strictly for informational purposes, and in no way should it be used as a substitute for consultation with your medical doctor or other health care professional. All facts in this book came from medical files, clinical journals, scientific publications, personal interviews, published trade books, self-published materials by experts, magazine articles, and the personal-practice experiences of the authorities quoted or sources cited. You should not consider educational material herein to be the practice of medicine or to replace consultation with a physician or other medical practitioner. The author and publisher are providing you with information in this work so that you can have the knowledge and can choose, at your own risk, to act on that knowledge. The author and publisher also urge all readers to be aware of their health status and to consult health professionals before beginning any health program, including changes in dietary habits.

Published by: Ulysses Press
            P.O. Box 3440
            Berkeley, CA 94703-3440

Library of Congress Catalog Card Number: 97-61589

ISBN: 1-56975-093-9

Printed in Canada by Best Book Manufacturers

First published as *Healing with Colour,* Gill & Macmillan, 1996

10 9 8 7 6 5 4 3 2 1

Editorial and production: Lily Chou
Typesetter: David Wells
Cover Design: B & L Design
Indexer: Sayre Van Young

Distributed in the United States by Publishers Group West and in Canada by Raincoast Books

TABLE OF CONTENTS

PART ONE

—

THE USES OF
COLOR IN HEALING

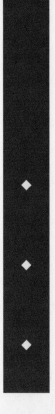

THE HISTORY OF HEALING WITH COLOR

"Let there be light: and there was light."
(Genesis 1:3)

In the early 1970s Lindsey, a friend of mine, took part in a unique experiment. With her husband, three young sons and ten other people, she was selected from several thousand applicants to live for twelve months in a reconstructed Iron Age settlement so that archaeologists, anthropologists and social historians could test various theories about patterns of living some 2000 years ago. Lindsey told me that one of the things she and her companions had missed most was color. Living in a dark hut in a small forest clearing had made them aware of color's importance to everyday life. They craved it so much that they attempted, unsuccessfully, to put some color into their drab lives by producing dyes.

Long-term hostages have also described a similar craving and their relief at being able to glimpse all the colors of the outside world.

Those who have never been deprived of color tend to take it for granted and generally don't realize its importance to our health and well-being. Nevertheless it is a basic need. Our early ancestors realized this, and the ancient healing traditions of many cultures reflect this awareness. The use of color in healing is not new. Color therapy, as it is now called, represents the rediscovery of some of the principles and practices known since the earliest times.

BECOMING ENLIGHTENED

For ancient man, light was seen as sustaining life and all the functions and processes of living things. "En-lightenment" was therefore synonymous with health in the literal sense of wholeness or holiness of body, mind and spirit. For the ancients, light was essentially a spiritual as well as a physical phenomenon.

Many ancient cultures worshipped the sun; the most important aim of life was for man to realize the light and thereby God. Ancient magic attempted to achieve this connection by "bringing down the light," transferring and reflecting its power. Magic and religion were thus inextricably linked with each other and with medicine.

LIGHT AND COLOR

Light is a narrow band of visible energy in the middle of a spectrum that embraces energies from cosmic rays to radio waves. These energies can be graded according to wavelength and measured in nanometers, each equivalent to one millionth of a millimeter. The spectrum of visible light falls within 380–760 nm. Each variation in wavelength within this band of energy can be sensed by our eyes and interpreted as a specific color. Reds have the longest wavelength, lowest frequency and least energy, while violets have the shortest wavelength, highest frequency and most energy. Beyond the red end of the visible spectrum are the longer wavelengths of infrared radiation, microwaves and radio waves; beyond the violet end are shorter wavelengths of ultraviolet radiation, X-rays, gamma rays and cosmic rays. The sun's energy produces all the wavelengths of color, from ultraviolet through the visual spectrum to infrared, in a roughly equal distribution. This is known as full-spectrum white light.

The effects of color on life must have been of great significance to early human beings, whose very existence was governed by light and darkness. Most living things appear to be vitalized by the bright reds, oranges and yellows of daylight and calmed and rejuvenated by the blues, indigos and violets of the night. For the ancients, the colors that make up sunlight were each considered to show a different aspect of the divine and to influence different qualities of life. Color is therefore an important feature in the symbolism of ancient cultures throughout the world, and the origins of healing with color in Western civilization can be traced back to the mythology of Ancient Egypt and Greece.

HEALING WITH COLOR IN THE ANCIENT WORLD

According to Ancient Egyptian mythology, the art of healing with color was founded by the god Thoth. He was known to the Ancient Greeks as Hermes Trismegistus, literally "Hermes thrice-greatest," because he was also credited with various works on mysticism and magic. Teachings attributed to him include the use of color in healing, and in the Hermetic tradition the Ancient Egyptians and Greeks used colored minerals, stones, crystals, salves and dyes as remedies, and painted treatment sanctuaries in various shades of color.

Interest in the physical nature of color developed in Ancient Greece alongside the concept of the elements — air, fire, water and earth. These fundamental constituents of the universe were associated with the qualities of coldness, heat, wetness and dryness, and also with four humors or bodily fluids — choler or yellow bile, (red) blood, (white) phlegm, and melancholy or black bile. These were thought to arise in four organs — the spleen, heart, liver and brain — and to determine emotional and physical disposition. Health involved the proper balance of these humors, and disease would result if their mixture was in an unbalanced proportion. Color was intrinsic to healing, which involved restoring the balance. Colored garments, oils, plasters, ointments and salves were used to treat disease.

By the end of the Classical period in Greece, these principles were included in the scientific framework that was to remain largely unchanged in the West until the Middle Ages. In the first century A.D., Aurelius Cornelius Celsus followed the doctrines established by Pythagoras and Hippocrates and included the use of colored ointments, plasters and flowers in several treatises on medicine.

HEALING WITH COLOR DURING THE MIDDLE AGES

With the coming of Christianity, however, all that was pagan was exorcised, including the healing practices of the Egyptians, Greeks and Romans. The progress of medicine throughout Europe was effectively halted while those who clung to traditional principles and practices of healing were persecuted. The ancient healing arts, preserved by secret oral tradition passed on to the initiates, thus became hidden or "occult."

It was an Arab physician and disciple of Aristotle, Avicenna (980–circa 1037), who advanced the art of healing. In his Canon of Medicine he made clear the vital importance of color in both diagnosis and treatment. Avicenna, noting that color was an observable symptom of disease, developed a chart which related color to temperament and the physical condition of the body. He used color in treatment, insisting that red moved the blood, blue or white cooled it, and yellow reduced pain and inflammation, prescribing potions of red flowers to cure blood disorders, and yellow flowers and morning sunlight to cure disorders of the biliary system.

Avicenna wrote also of the possible dangers of color in treatment, observing that a person with a nosebleed, for example, should not gaze at things of a brilliant red color or be exposed to red light because this would stimulate the sanguineous humor, whereas blue would soothe it and reduce blood flow.

The Renaissance saw a resurgence in the art of healing in Europe. One of the most renowned healers of the period was Theophrastus Bombastus von Hohenheim (1493–1541), known as Paracelsus, who attributed his understanding of the laws and practices of medicine to his conversations with witches (women who were primarily pagan healers purged by the Church).

Paracelsus regarded light and color as essential for good health and used them extensively in treatment, together with elixirs, charms and talismans, herbs and minerals. A great exponent of alchemy, Paracelsus insisted that its true purpose was not to make gold but to prepare effective medicines, and he used liquid gold to treat ailments of all kinds, apparently with a good deal of success. Consequently his fame as a great physician spread throughout Europe.

ENLIGHTENMENT, SCIENCE AND HEALING

However, after the Middle Ages Paracelsus and other alchemists lost their prestige when mysticism and magic were overtaken by rationalism and science. By the eighteenth century, "enlightenment" had taken on a new meaning. It was the name given to a philosophical movement that stressed the importance of reason and the critical appraisal of existing ideas. Reason dictated that all knowledge had to be certain and evident; anything about which there could be doubt was rejected. As a result the divine gradually disappeared from the scientific world view.

By the nineteenth century the emphasis in science was exclusively on the material rather than the spiritual. As medicine came under the umbrella of science it, too, focused on the material physical body, ignoring the mind and spirit. With the advent of physical medicine and such treatments as surgery and antiseptics, interest in healing with color declined. It didn't resurface until the nineteenth century, and then not in Europe but North America.

In 1876, Augustus Pleasanton published *Blue and Sun-lights*, in which he reported his findings on the effects of color in plants, animals and humans. He claimed that the quality, yield and size of grapes could be significantly increased if they were grown in greenhouses made with alternating blue and transparent panes of glass. He also reported having cured certain diseases and increased fertility as well as the rate of physical maturation in animals by exposing them to blue light. In addition, Pleasanton maintained that blue light was effective in treating human disease and pain. His work gained supporters but was dismissed by the medical establishment as unscientific.

However, in 1877 a distinguished physician named Dr. Seth Pancoast published *Blue and Red Lights*, in which he, too, advocated the use of color in healing.

Edwin Babbit's *The Principles of Light and Color* was published in 1878; the second edition, published in 1896, attracted worldwide attention. Babbit advanced a comprehensive theory of healing with color. He identified the color red as a stimulant, notably of blood and to a lesser extent to the nerves; yellow and orange as nerve stimulants; blue and violet as soothing to all systems and with anti-inflammatory properties. Accordingly, Babbit prescribed red for paralysis, consumption, physical exhaustion and chronic rheumatism; yellow as a laxative, emetic and purgative, and for bronchial difficulties; and blue for inflammatory conditions, sciatica, meningitis, nervous headache, irritability and sunstroke. Babbit developed various devices, including a special cabinet called the Thermolume, which used colored glass and natural light to produce colored light; and the Chromo Disk, a funnel-shaped device fitted with special color filters that could localize light onto various parts of the body.

Babbit established the correspondence between colors and minerals, which he used as an addition to treatment with colored light, and developed elixirs by irradiating water with sunlight filtered through colored lenses. He claimed that this "potentized" water retained the energy of the vital elements within the particular color filter used, and that it had remarkable healing power. Solar tinctures of this kind are still made and used today by many color therapists.

Chromopaths then sprang up throughout the country and Britain, developing extensive color prescriptions for every conceivable ailment. By the end of the nineteenth century, red light was used to prevent scars from forming in cases of smallpox, and startling cures were later reported among tuberculosis patients exposed to sunlight and ultraviolet rays. Nevertheless, the medical profession remained skeptical of claims made about healing with color.

TWENTIETH-CENTURY SCIENCE AND HEALING WITH COLOR

Investigations into the therapeutic use of color were carried out in Europe during the early twentieth century, notably by Rudolph Steiner, who related color to form, shape and sound. He suggested that the vibrational quality of certain colors is amplified by some forms, and that certain combinations of color and shape have either destructive or regenerative effects on living organisms. In the schools inspired by Steiner's work, classrooms are painted and textured to correspond to the "mood" of children at various stages of their development.

Rudolph Steiner's work was continued by Theo Gimbel, who established the Hygeia Studios and College of Color Therapy in Britain. Among the principles explored by Gimbel are the claims of Max Lüscher, a former professor of psychology at Basle University, who claimed that color preferences demonstrate states of mind and/or glandular imbalance and can be used as the basis for physical and psychological diagnosis. Lüscher's theory, which forms the basis of the Lüscher Color Test, rests on the idea that the significance of color for man originates in his early history, when his behavior was governed by night and day. Lüscher believed that the colors associated with these two environments — yellow and dark blue — are connected with differences in metabolic rate and glandular secretions appropriate to the energy required for nighttime sleep and daytime hunting. He also believed that autonomic (involuntary) responses are associated with other colors.

Support for Lüscher's theories was provided in the 1940s by the Russian scientist S. V. Krakov, who established that the color red stimulates the sympathetic part of the autonomic nervous system, while blue stimulates the parasympathetic part. His findings were confirmed in 1958 by Robert Gerard.

Gerard found that red produced feelings of arousal and was disturbing to anxious or tense subjects, while blue generated feelings of tranquility and well-being and had a calming effect. The discovery that blood pressure increases under red light and decreases under blue light led Gerard to suggest that psychophysiological activation increases with wavelength from blue to red.

Although cautious about his findings and insisting on the need for further research, Gerard highlighted the possible therapeutic benefits of the color blue and recommended it as supplementary therapy in the treatment of various conditions. Among other suggestions, Gerard pointed to the possible uses of blue as a tranquilizer and relaxant in anxious individuals and as a way of reducing blood pressure in the treatment of hypertension.

Dr. Harry Wohlfarth also showed that certain colors have measurable and predictable effects on the autonomic nervous system of people. In numerous studies, he found that blood pressure, pulse and respiration rates increase most under yellow light, moderately under orange and minimally under red, while decreasing most under black, moderately under blue and minimally under green.

Subsequent research on plants and animals conducted by the photobiologist Dr. John Ott demonstrated the effects of color on growth and development. Plants grown under red glass were found to shoot up four times quicker than those grown in ordinary sunlight, and to grow much more slowly under green glass. However, although red light initially overstimulated plants, their growth was subsequently stunted, whereas blue light produced slower growth initially but taller, thicker plants later.

Rodents kept under blue plastic grew normally, but when kept under red or pink plastic their appetite and growth rate increased. If kept under blue light animals grew denser coats.

During the 1950s, studies suggested that neonatal jaundice, a potentially fatal condition found in two-thirds of premature babies, could be successfully treated by exposure to sunlight. This was confirmed in the 1960s, and white light replaced the high-risk blood transfusions in the treatment of this condition. Blue light was later found to be more effective and less hazardous than full-spectrum light (the most common form of treatment for neonatal jaundice).

Bright white full-spectrum light is also now being used in the treatment of cancers, SAD (seasonal affective disorder, so-called "winter depression"), anorexia, bulimia nervosa, insomnia, jet lag, shift-working, alcohol and drug dependency and to reduce overall levels of medication.

The blue light found to be successful in the treatment of neo-natal jaundice has also been shown to be effective in the treatment of rheumatoid arthritis. In studies by S. F. McDonald, most of those exposed to blue light for variable periods up to fifteen minutes experienced a significant degree of pain relief. It was concluded that the pain reduction was directly related both to the blue light and the length of exposure to it. Blue light is also used in healing injured tissue and preventing scar tissue, in the treatment of cancers and non-malignant tumors, as well as skin and lung conditions.

In 1990, scientists reported to the annual conference of the American Association for the Advancement of Science on the successful use of blue light in the treatment of a wide variety of psychological problems, including addictions, eating disorders, impotence and depression.

RECENT APPLICATIONS OF COLOR TO HEALING

At the other end of the color spectrum, red light has been shown to be effective in the treatment of migraine headaches and cancer. As a result, color is becoming widely accepted as a therapeutic tool with various medical applications. A new technique which has been developed over the past two decades as a result of pioneering research is photodynamic therapy, or PDT. This is based on the discovery that certain intravenously injected photosensitive chemicals not only accumulate in cancer cells but selectively identify these cells under ultraviolet light. These photosensitive chemicals then exclusively destroy the cancer cells when activated by red light, whose longer wavelength allows it to penetrate tissue more deeply than other colors. PDT can be used for both diagnosis and treatment. Dr. Thomas Dougherty, who developed PDT, reports that in a worldwide experiment more than 3000 people with a wide variety of malignant tumors have been successfully treated with this technique.

Other Therapeutic Applications of Color

Color is also used therapeutically in a variety of nonmedical settings. In some cases its effects have been quite accidental, as in a report to me by the governor of a newly built prison in which each of its four wings had been painted a different color. Both he and his staff found that the behavior of the prisoners varied significantly depending on which wing they lived in, although their allocation to each had been random. Those in red and yellow wings were more inclined to violence than those in the blue and green wings.

Experimental research lends support to these observations. Viewing red light has been found to increase subjects' strength by 13.5 percent and to elicit 5.8 percent more electrical activity in the arm muscles. For this reason it is now used to improve the performance of athletes. Whereas red light appears to help athletes who need short, quick bursts of energy, blue light assists in performances requiring a more steady energy output.

By comparison, pink has been found to have a tranquilizing and calming effect within minutes of exposure. It suppresses hostile, aggressive and anxious behavior — interesting given its traditional association with women in Western culture. Pink holding cells are now widely used to reduce violent and aggressive behavior among prisoners, and some sources have reported a reduction of muscle strength in inmates within 2.7 seconds. It appears that when in pink surroundings people cannot be aggressive even if they want to because the color saps their energy.

By contrast, yellow should be avoided in such contexts because it is highly stimulating. Gimbel has suggested a possible relationship between violent street crime and sodium yellow street lighting.

Research has also shown that color-tinted eyeglasses can be highly effective in the treatment of learning difficulties, notably dyslexia. This was first discovered by psychologist Helen Irlen, but was regarded sceptically until recent investigations by the British Medical Research Council confirmed Irlen's claims. In June 1993, a new optician's device called the Intuitive Colorimeter was made available to British opticians so they could measure which tint — bright pink, yellow, green or blue — best helps people who normally see text as swirling, wobbling or with letters appearing in the wrong order.

CONTEMPORARY UNDERSTANDING OF THE PHYSICAL EFFECTS OF COLOR

Until recently, the function of light was thought to relate largely to sight. However, it is now well established that color need not actually be seen for it to have definite psychological and physiological effects. It can also be distinguished by blind, colorblind and blindfolded subjects. This phenomenon, referred to as eyeless sight, dermo-optic vision or bio-introscopy, has been researched since the 1920s, when it was established that hypnotized blindfolded subjects could recognize colors and shapes with their foreheads, and that nonhypnotized blindfolded subjects could precisely describe colors and shapes presented under glass.

Research in Russia during the 1960s was stimulated by studies of Roza Kulesheva, who, when blindfolded, could distinguish color and shape with her fingertips, and could also read this way. Other experiments found that Kulesheva was not exceptional; one in six experimental subjects could recognize color with their fingertips after only 20–30 minutes training, and blind people developed this sensitivity even more quickly.

Some subjects who could distinguish color correctly by holding their fingers 20–80 centimeters above color cards described experiencing sensations varying from needle pricks to faint breezes, depending on the color. Even when heat differences, structural differences in dyestuffs and other variables were controlled, people were still able to distinguish colors accurately, whether they were put under glass, tracing paper, aluminium foil, brass or copper plates. The phenomenon remains something of a puzzle.

Understanding of these effects has come about only as a result of research into the hormones melatonin and serotonin, both of which are produced by the pineal gland in the brain. Melatonin is known to be the crucial chemical pathway by which animals respond to light and synchronize their bodily functioning with diurnal, lunar and seasonal variations. Serotonin is a very important neurotransmitter in the brain, whose action has been linked with mental disturbances such as schizophrenia and hallucinogenic states.

Serotonin, a stimulant, is produced by day, whereas the output of melatonin — which is linked with sleep — increases when it is dark and has a generally depressive effect. This is reversed when it is light and production of melatonin drops. Its main site of action appears to be the hypothalamus, the part of the brain involved in mediating the effects of various hormones and regulating emotions. However, changes in the output of melatonin in response to light influence every cell of the body, notably the reproductive processes, which are very sensitive to such variations. Very high levels of melatonin have been found in women with ovulation problems and anorexia nervosa (a characteristic feature of which is amenorrhoea, or absence of periods) in men with low sperm count, and people suffering from seasonal affective disorder (SAD), which usually occurs during winter.

Depression in general appears to be closely linked with melatonin levels, and sufferers tend to show rapid improvement in response to natural sunlight or light therapy using full-spectrum lamps. Research has also confirmed that certain parts of the brain are not only light sensitive but actually respond differently to different wavelengths; it is now believed that different wavelengths (color) of radiation interact differently with the endocrine system to stimulate or reduce hormone production.

It might be thought that modern-day healing with color is based on the discoveries of Western science over the past few decades. However, it is based on an altogether more ancient and esoteric science whose principles and practices have yet to be acknowledged, much less verified by Western scientists. Healing with color is rooted in ancient mysticism, the major principles of which are common to many different cultures throughout the world.

2

THE PRINCIPLES OF
HEALING WITH COLOR

"You are light."
(Luke 11:34)

In mystic traditions, all objects — living or not —
are seen as possessing other bodies invisible to
normal sight. These envelop the physical body
and act as a medium for the interplay of subtle
energies in the immediate environment. St. Paul
expressed such a view, claiming that "there is a
natural body and a physical body" (Corinthians
15:44). The former was called a halo by early
Christians and shown as a hazy colored light en-
veloping the entire body. In later Renaissance and
medieval art it was confined to the head region.

Variously referred to as the Ka in Ancient Egypt;
the aura in Ancient Greece; the döppelganger in
medieval Europe; the vital body in certain Rosi-
crucian schools; the astral, etheric body or double
in other Western occult traditions; the *perispirit* in

French spiritism; and the *linga sharirah* in the East, this phenomenon was considered synonymous with the spirit or soul, and as surviving death. Together, these individual energy bodies were thought to make up the universal energy field.

Traditional Views of the Human Energy Field

Mystics consider that subtle energies from the environment are distributed through the body by way of several major power centers on the surface of the nonphysical counterpart, or energy body. These are described as three-dimensional pulsating vortices that appear to seers or clairvoyants like funnels, trumpets or convolvulus flowers, and rotate rhythmically from the midpoint outward rather like pinwheels. According to the direction of spin, the wheels either draw energy into or direct it out of the body, vitalizing or enervating it.

Much was written about these centers in Ancient Hindu texts. The Theosophists, who first wrote about them in English in the late nineteenth and early twentieth centuries, retained the Sanskrit term *chakra*, meaning wheel, to refer to them. Early European mystics were also familiar with them, and ancient knowledge of the chakras in the West is suggested in the symbolism of Ancient Egyptian monuments and Freemasonry. Similar ideas are found in the traditional wisdom of North and Central American Indians, the Eskimo and the Tibetans. Within these different traditions, though, the number and location of the chakras vary.

The Chakras

The Hindu texts locate seven major chakras along the vertical axis of the energy body, corresponding with the spine in the physical body and a number of minor chakras elsewhere on its surface. According to ancient wisdom, energy in the form of light is drawn into the body's immaterial counterpart,

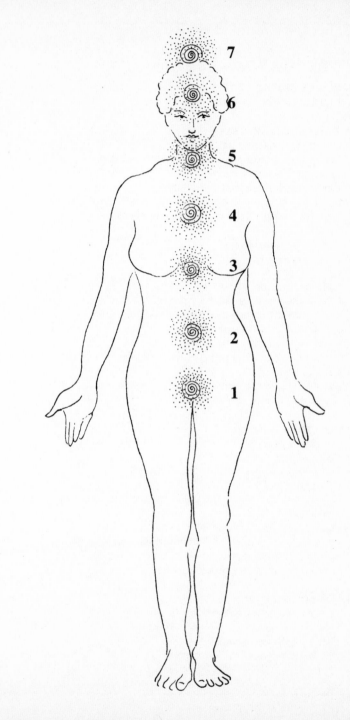

Key to illustration:

1. Base Chakra
Location: base of the spine
Color: red
Endocrine: ovaries, testes
Oils: myrrh, vetivert, patchouli
Gems/Minerals: ruby, garnet, bloodstone, red jasper, smoky quartz, black tourmaline
Foods: proteins, red fruits/vegetables
Positive Qualities: security, grounding, stability, health, courage
Negative Qualities: self-centeredness, insecurity, anger, violence

2. Navel Chakra (Hara)
Location: navel area
Color: orange
Endocrine: adrenal glands
Oils: sandalwood, cardamom, ginger
Gems/Minerals: carnelian, coral, gold calcite, amber, citrine, gold topaz, peach aventurine
Foods: yellow fruits/vegetables
Positive Qualities: gut instincts, emotions, sexuality, exercise, movement
Negative Qualities: overindulgence, sexual difficulties, envy, bladder/uterine disorders

3. Solar Plexus Chakra
Location: approximately two inches above the navel
Color: yellow
Endocrine: pancreas, adrenal glands, liver
Oils: lemon, citronella
Gems/Minerals: citrine, gold, gold topaz, amber, tiger's eye, gold calcite
Foods: yellow fruits/vegetables
Positive Qualities: intellect, rationality, will, personal power
Negative Qualities: abuse of power, anger, fear, hate, stress disorders, digestive problems

4. Heart Chakra
Location: center of the chest
Color: green
Endocrine: thymus gland
Oils: pine, bergamot, invila, melissa

Gems/Minerals: emerald, beryl, green tourmaline, jade, agate,
   malachite, green aventurine, rose quartz, rhodochrosite
Foods: green fruits/vegetables
Positive Qualities: unconditional love, compassion, forgiveness,
   understanding, balance, openness, touch, sensitivity, immunity
Negative Qualities: resentment, insensitivity, imbalance, heart
   and circulation problems, rheumatism

5. Throat Chakra
Location: center of the throat
Color: sky blue
Endocrine: thyroid gland
Oils: lavender, chamomile, geranium
Gems/Minerals: turquoise, crysocolla, blue topaz, sodalite, lapis
   lazuli, aquamarine, kyanite
Foods: blue fruit/vegetables, asparagus
Positive Qualities: speech, communication, creative expression
Negative Qualities: speech and communication problems,
   thyroid dysfunction

6. Brow Chakra (Third Eye)
Location: center of the forehead
Color: indigo (dark blue)
Endocrine: pineal gland
Oils: patchouli, frankincense
Gems/Minerals: lapis lazuli, azuri, sodalite, sapphire
Foods: purple/blue fruits/vegetables
Positive Qualities: soul realization, intuition, insight,
   imagination, clairvoyance, concentration
Negative Qualities: lack of concentration, cynicism, headaches,
   bad dreams, detachment from reality

7. Crown Chakra
Location: top of the head
Color: violet
Endocrine: pituitary gland
Oils: elemi, frankincense
Gems/Minerals: amethyst, alexandrite, sugalite, purple fluorite,
   selenite
Foods: purple fruits/vegetables
Positive Qualities: union with higher self, the infinite,
   spirituality, higher consciousness
Negative Qualities: alienation, despair, confusion

which acts as a prism, breaking it down into seven streams corresponding with the frequency bands of the color spectrum. Each of these is drawn through resonance to a chakra whose vibrations are of the same frequency. These vibrations become progressively more dense, heavy and lower in frequency along the vertical axis of the body. At its base they merge with and arise from earth energies, represented in Indian thought as a coiled serpent — Kundalini — and in Chinese thought by a dragon. The upward spiral motion of these energies around the central axis of the spine is also represented in the caduceus, the traditional symbol of the healing arts in Ancient Greece, which is still retained as the emblem of modern Western medicine.

The chakras, which may be thought of as transmitters or transformers of energy, are believed to vibrate at a characteristic frequency as they distribute energy throughout the body. The energy patterns around each chakra, although always changing, are mostly of a certain color whose vibrations correspond with its basic frequency. The prevailing color of a chakra indicates how well its energies are being transformed and transmitted at a given time and therefore reflect current experience.

In ancient traditions, each chakra is also associated with a musical note, a symbolic form and certain elements of the same characteristic vibrational frequency (which vary according to the tradition). Certain traditions also assign planets to the chakras, suggesting that they are sensitive to planetary influence, thus providing a physical basis for astrology. Recently the chakras have also been associated with the location and functioning of the major nerve plexuses of the body, each of which is connected to one of the glands of the endocrine system; the slightest imbalance of energy in any chakra is thought to influence the corresponding gland, giving rise to fluctuations in hormones that are secreted directly into the bloodstream, producing immediate changes in mood, appearance, tension, respiration, digestion, intuition and intelligence. The correct and balanced action of these seven chakras is expressed as absolute and perfect health on all levels.

The principal features of the human chakra system common to many traditions are as follows.

The first, root or base chakra, known in Sanskrit as *Muladhara* and located at a position corresponding with the base of the spine, is the first manifestation of the life force in the physical body. Its functioning determines the person's level of physical energy and the will to live in physical reality. It is concerned with basic survival and physical health; being intimately connected with the prostate and testes in men and the uterus in women, it influences sexual activity and regulates creativity. This energy primarily affects the legs, the hip joints and base of the spine, overlapping into the pelvic area, providing the strength to support the physical body and influencing safety and security. However, the coccyx functions on the etheric level as a pump, directing the flow of energy up the spine and connecting each chakra with the life force.

Psychologically, the first chakra is associated with feelings of being securely grounded, "well rooted" and belonging. It is thought to be mostly red, influenced by Saturn, associated with the element earth, the symbolic form of the square, the metal lead (base metal), the sense of smell and the sound vibration LA. (The symbols and sounds included here and below are from the Tantric tradition.)

The second or navel chakra, Svadhistana, located in the pelvic region midway between the pubis and the navel, is considered in traditional systems to be the center of sexual activity. Because sexuality is an expression of the life force this chakra is closely related to the base chakra and influences physical and sexual vitality. It is situated in the region referred to as the gut or belly, which the Japanese term the *hara*, and is associated with the liver, pancreas, spleen, kidneys and bladder, and therefore with metabolism, digestion, detoxification, immunity to disease, and the balance of fluids and sugars within the body. It is also thought to have glandular connections with the testes and ovaries, and to influence the production of the hormones testosterone and estrogen.

On the psychological level it relates to passions or "gut feelings" and emotions, and to issues people care deeply about — power, sex and material wealth. It is associated with the color orange, the influence of Jupiter, water, tin, the sense of taste, the symbolic form of a pyramid with its capstone removed, and the sound BA.

The third or solar plexus chakra, Manipura, positioned slightly above the navel, is thought of as the center of personal power or the power to act, and therefore with the sense of vision. It is associated with the adrenal glands, which through the production of adrenalin profoundly affect the sympathetic nervous system and thereby muscular energy, heartbeat, digestion, circulation and mood.

Traditionally it is related to mental functioning — the intellect or rational mind, intentionality and will — but it is also directly related to the second chakra and emotional life. Thought to be primarily yellow, it is associated with Mars, fire, iron, sight, the symbolic form of the circle, and the sound RA.

The fourth or heart chakra, Anahata, found in the center of the chest over the breast bone, is believed to relate to the thymus gland situated behind the sternum, the main function of which in adults is to create immunity to disease. Traditionally it is associated with love and compassion, feeling, sensitivity, touch, the skin and the hands, and the color green. Interestingly it is known that many of the body's immune cells are located in the skin and can be stimulated by touch.

It is thought to be influenced by Venus, associated with air, copper, the symbol of the equilateral cross, and the two-syllable sound YA Mn.

The fifth or throat chakra, Vishuddhi, located at the front of the throat, is thought to influence the thyroid gland, which affects the metabolism, musculature and thermoregulation of the body. Traditionally it relates to communication and self-expression, to hearing and taking responsibility for one's personal needs. It is associated with sky blue, the planet Mercury, ether, hearing, the symbolic form of the chalice, and the sound HA.

The sixth or brow chakra, Ajna, found just above and between the eyebrows in the center of the forehead, is traditionally known as the "third eye" and is identified with visual imagery, insight, intuitive understanding, clairvoyance, psychic abilities and ecstasy. It is associated with the pineal gland, which according to contemporary research has a significant role in processing mental imagery and unconscious processes, and is also responsible for the production of the hormones melatonin and serotonin. Its color is midnight blue or indigo, and its symbols are the moon, gold and silver, the six-pointed star, and the sound AH.

The seventh or crown chakra, Sahasrara, is positioned in the center of the upper skull; traditionally regarded as the seat of the soul, it is identified with pure or enlightened being, spirituality and integration of the whole being. It is associated with the pituitary, the master endocrine gland, which regulates the functioning of the other glands, and is closely associated with the pineal gland. Its color is purple or violet, symbolized by the thousand-petaled lotus, and the sacred sound OM (oh aa um), which is considered to be the total amalgam of all sound and of all creation.

According to the chakra system, human beings have a seven-fold nature. The first and second chakras are mostly concerned with receiving and distributing physical energies, and combine to give a person potency, virility and the will to live. The third, fourth and fifth chakras are concerned with psychological energies and therefore with personality rather than physical traits; the sixth and seventh chakras are concerned with spiritual energies that are an expression of the individual's relationship to his or her spirit or soul.

The chakras function as an integrated system rather than in isolation. If one begins to malfunction, so will others as they attempt to compensate for reduced energy transmission in one center by working overtime. The chakra system thus provides the impetus for the regulated, balanced flow of energy throughout the whole person which is necessary for health.

THE AURA

Traditionally the flow of energy is not confined within the physical body as we normally thought of it. In the ancient view, the body emits a radiant energy that relates specifically to the location and intensity of energy within it, and therefore reveals something about how it is functioning.

This three-dimensional emanation, which surrounds the body in all directions and extends for some distance beyond its surface, is widely referred to as the aura, and represents the sum total of the energy emitted by the chakras.

Normally invisible but discernible by seers and clairvoyants — who since the earliest times have described it as a large shimmering oval, comprising a mass of fine bright fibers or rays arranged in seven bands, each corresponding to the functioning of a chakra — the aura reveals the physical, psychological and spiritual well-being of the person it envelops.

When the chakras are functioning normally, each will "open" by spinning clockwise and drawing energy in from the universal energy field to distribute throughout the body. When

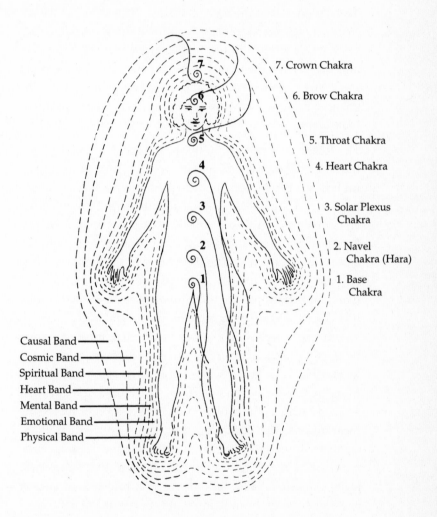

7. Crown Chakra

6. Brow Chakra

5. Throat Chakra

4. Heart Chakra

3. Solar Plexus
Chakra

2. Navel
Chakra (Hara)

1. Base
Chakra

Causal Band
Cosmic Band
Spiritual Band
Heart Band
Mental Band
Emotional Band
Physical Band

*A two-dimensional representation of the human aura showing
each band as it relates to specific chakras*

the transmission of energy has occurred, the color originating from each should be very pale and translucent.

However, when the chakra spins counterclockwise it remains closed to incoming energies, which consequently are not distributed within the body and show themselves as darker, denser patches or blotches of color in the aura. The space between the body and the first color emanation of the aura is referred to as the ovum. It is not "empty" as such, being the densest and therefore most easily visible part of the energy field, but is colorless or a dull white/gold, appearing to be blank.

The first layer of the aura, the health band, emanates from the base chakra and reflects the overall vitality of the physical body. It is traditionally described in metaphysical literature as red. The second band of the aura, known as the emotional or astral band, emanates from the second chakra. It reflects physical and sexual activity, and "gut feelings," and is orange in color. The third layer of the aura, the mental band, comes from the solar plexus chakra and reflects mental functions based on the intellect and personal power. It is yellow, and shiny or brilliant in a mentally alive person. The fourth layer of the aura, or heart band, emanates from the heart chakra. It is green and reflects inspiration in all forms. The fifth layer of the aura, or causal band, comes from the throat chakra and is blue, reflecting self-expression and the karma of the soul — its progress through successive incarnations. The dark blue sixth layer, or spiritual band, emanates from the sixth chakra, reflecting the person's spiritual development and intuitive awareness; and the seventh layer, or cosmic band, reflects the soul principle or cosmic consciousness of the individual. It is purple in color.

Each band radiates different colors of varying intensity that reveal to those who can discern them the person's state of health, character, emotional disposition and tendencies, abilities, attitudes, past problems and spiritual development.

The aura can therefore be used for diagnosis; throughout history seers (or sensitives) have reported using it as a basis for healing.

A study of orthodox Western physicians has also revealed that many diagnose illness through the energy field they perceive around their patients or through the energy vortices connected with the endocrine system. One practitioner, John Pierrakos, has conducted extensive research on the phenomenon.

SCIENTIFIC MEASUREMENT OF THE CHAKRA–AURA SYSTEM

While the vital force is self-evident to many healers, it has eluded scientific measurement until recently. This may be because its subtle energies can only react with and be detected by living organisms. When it finds its counterpart in a living being, a detectable reaction results. This, it is claimed, is the basis for healing diagnoses, dowsing and water divining. However, because this force is not easily detected by physical instruments in the orthodox scientific world, it is deemed to have no physical reality.

That science is blinded by the limitations of its own tools is clear from the history of Western research into the human energy field during this century. In 1911, Dr. Walter Kilner of St. Thomas' Hospital, London, developed a special kind of glass which he claimed allowed the aura to be seen objectively. This — and his prediction that it would in the future be possible to photograph the aura and use it for more accurate diagnosis of all kinds of illness — was dismissed as fanciful. The views of Dr. F. S. C. Northrup of Yale, who proposed the existence of dynamic life fields around living things, were similarly rejected, as was the discovery of an energy body possessed by all human beings claimed by Yale professor of anatomy, H. S. Burr.

However, during the 1930s developments in high voltage photography by Russian scientists Semyon and Valentina

Kirlian, which revealed streams of apparent energy flowing from the fingertips in a manner suggested by traditional aura theory, appeared to fulfill Kilner's predictions. Over the next ten years the Kirlians became convinced that these energy streams reflected the well-being or otherwise of an organism, and this view subsequently gained support from research on plants. During the 1960s, another Russian researcher, Leonidov, developed a lightless microphoto that provided further objective evidence for the aura.

Professor Vladimir Inyushin, who developed the Kirlians' research, subsequently described the energy field around living forms as a biological plasma body, claiming — as Burr had done previously — that this is a whole unified organism emitting its own electromagnetic fields, which are the basis of all biological fields.

The chakras have also been the subject of considerable scientific research, most notably by the Japanese Professor Hiroshi Motoyama. Commencing his research in the 1960s with studies of psychics and healers, Motoyama developed various sophisticated physiological devices to measure subtle energies in and around the body. He devised an instrument to determine experimentally the working of the chakras. It measures the electromagnetic fields around the body, and can show, by subtle changes in these, when a chakra is naturally active or activated by some other means. Motoyama concluded that the energy systems underpinning traditional Chinese and Indian medicine are fundamentally the same, despite differences in terminology.

Until recently much of this pioneering scientific research into the subtle energies of the chakras and aura took place only in Russia and the East. There is now an increasing interest in subtle body and energy systems here in the West. Professor Thelma Moss of the Neuropsychiatric Institute of the University of California School of Medicine was the first serious researcher of these phenomena in this country. Since her pioneering work there have been intensive investigations of these energy systems, most notably at the University of California by Dr. Valerie Hunt. In Britain, Professor Dennis Milner at Birmingham University has conducted research into Kirlian photography, and the psychophysiology of the chakra system has been mapped out by Dr. Serena Roney-Dougal.

THE CHAKRA–AURA SYSTEM AND HEALTH

In North America and Canada there has been extensive investigation of clairvoyants such as Jack Schwarz and Rosaline Bruyère, who perceive chakra and aura energies and use them in diagnosis and treatment. This research appears to confirm the observations of the ancients.

Disturbances in the energy distribution of the base chakra are found to correspond with lack of physical energy and general ill-health, chronic lower back pain, sciatica, varicose veins and rectal problems — including tumors and cancerous growths.

Energy blockages in the second chakra are generally associated with reduced physical and sexual activity because the pelvic area is the major source of vitality in the body. Imbalances in this chakra are commonly found in women with problems such as menstrual difficulties, infertility, vaginal infections, ovarian cysts, endometriosis, tumors and cancers of the female organs; and in men with impotence and prostate problems. In both men and women pelvic and lower back pain, sexual difficulties and disease, slipped discs, bladder and urinary problems, and frequent loss of sexual fluids commonly occur when this chakra is unstable.

The most common physical conditions associated with disturbances in the energy flow of the third or solar plexus chakra include: arthritis; ulcers and related stomach problems — poor digestion, chronic or acute indigestion; eating disorders such as anorexia and bulimia nervosa; nausea;

abnormal appetite; colon and intestinal problems including cancer, pancreatitis and pancreatic cancer; diabetes; kidney and liver problems; hepatitis; gallbladder and adrenal gland disorders; and influenza.

When the fourth, or heart, chakra is unstable there may be cardiac or circulatory abnormalities which commonly result in: heart attack; enlarged heart; congestive heart failure; blocked arteries; asthma; allergies; lung problems including cancer, bronchial difficulties and pneumonia; poor circulation; and upper back and shoulder problems.

People with imbalances in the fifth or throat chakra have a tendency toward skin problems and allergies, and as a result of poor detoxification within the body: thyroid conditions, throat infections, sore throat, loss of voice, laryngitis, tonsillitis, cancers of the throat and mouth, problems with the teeth and gums, misalignment of the jaw, curved spine, stiff neck, tension headaches arising from the base of the neck, and swollen glands.

The sixth chakra, or "third eye," is thought to exert a strong influence on the balanced functioning of the endocrine system, visual functioning, sleep, clarity of mental functions and general energy levels. Instability in this chakra is reflected in: fatigue and tiredness, migraine and tension headache, irritability, anxiety, nervousness and depression, nervous breakdown, psychotic illness including schizophrenia, sleep irregularities, coma, neurological disorders including blindness and deafness, epilepsy and seizures, learning difficulties, brain tumors, stroke and blood clots to the brain.

Instability in the seventh or crown chakra can result in disorders of the nervous system, paralysis, bone problems and debilitating illnesses such as multiple sclerosis.

Taken together, the chakra and aura systems provide a comprehensive and consistent account of the distribution and functioning of subtle energies within and around the body, and a framework for what can be thought of as subtle energy therapies such as those traditionally practiced in India, Tibet, China, Japan, among American Indians, Aboriginals and the Kahunas of Hawaii. These include age-old practices such as acupuncture, acupressure or Shiatsu, Ayurvedic medicine, and healing with color; and more recent practices such as reflexology, cranio-sacral therapy, radionics, polarity therapy and homeopathy.

All of these healing systems view disease as fundamentally spiritual in origin, as an imbalance in the energies of the soul which initially shows itself as a conflict or problem at the psychological level and only finally as symptoms of physical illness. These approaches to healing therefore address disease primarily at the spiritual and psychological level, and diagnosis tends to focus on these aspects rather than the physical.

DIAGNOSING DISORDER THROUGH THE AURA AND CHAKRAS

Physicist and healer Barbara Ann Brennan believes that auric diagnosis is especially helpful because "the aura is really the 'missing link' between biology and physical medicine and psychotherapy. It is the 'place' where all emotions, thoughts, memories and behavior patterns are located," and reflects the activity of the chakras, which represent the psychological patterns evolving in a person's life throughout their development. Brennan observes that most people react to unpleasant experiences by blocking their feelings. This affects the chakras by restricting much of their energy flow, and inhibits fully balanced psychological functioning. If a child is rejected many times when she tries to give love to others, she will probably stop trying to do so and will consequently repress the inner feelings of love on which her former actions were based. To do this she has to stop or slow down the energy flow through the heart chakra, which in turn will affect its functioning. It may become blocked with stagnant energy, spin irregularly or counterclockwise, become distorted or eventually result in the development of a physical problem. This same process applies to all the chakras.

CHAKRA DYSFUNCTION AND PSYCHOLOGICAL DISORDER

Brennan and Pierrakos have related chakra dysfunction to psychological disorder, and their analysis generally agrees with traditional and more contemporary accounts, the common points of which can be found below.

When the base chakra is functioning normally, you are well-grounded in the here-and-now of physical reality, and have power and vitality or presence, and a strong will to live. You feel secure and grounded. When this chakra is blocked you lack physical vitality and strength, and fail to make a strong impression in the physical world. You lack "presence," are insecure in and threatened by the world, may not feel at home anywhere, and feel alone and unsupported. Motoyama's research reveals that a predominance of energy in this chakra can lead to violent aggression, and that accidents causing sudden injury to the coccyx — the spinal energy pump — can cause an uncontrolled release of energy that may contribute to certain types of psychosis.

Normal functioning of the second or sacral chakra is related to giving and receiving physical and sexual pleasure, the capacity for orgasm, and to strong gut feelings and emotions. However, if the center is dysfunctional, you will have sexual difficulties, feelings of sexual inadequacy, impotence, lack of orgasm, feelings of low self-esteem and general anxiety. This chakra has also been associated with a passion for money and power. So when it is not working properly, your anxiety about money, material possessions and power may create imbalances in all forms of relationship with the material world. The opening of this chakra is also associated with intuition, uncontrolled psychokinetic phenomena such as poltergeist activity and the development of extrasensory perception such as precognition and out-of-body experiences.

The third or solar plexus chakra normally empowers a person mentally and emotionally. When it is unstable you may have rapid mood swings, a tendency toward depression and anger at feeling controlled by others, a tendency to victimize and to be highly critical of people, and a fear of failure. If underfunctioning, this chakra gives rise to anxiety and feelings of disempowerment and submissiveness; if over-functioning it may create aggression and domination of others. Energy dysfunctions in this chakra often result in stress disorders, characterized by excessive adrenaline production, ulcers, nervous disorders or chronic fatigue. When it is blocked, feeling and thinking will not be very clear, decision making will be poor and you may fear taking responsibility for your life, thoughts, feelings, attitudes and personal actions. Clairvoyance and mental telepathy may accompany the opening of this chakra.

The more open the fourth or heart chakra, the greater a person's capacity to love becomes. When functioning well you feel self-love and love for family, friends, children, animals, nature and all life forms on earth. If this chakra is dysfunctional you may be overexcitable, extroverted and ambitious for fame. When blocked, other people may be seen as obstacles to accomplishment and fulfillment of your heart's desires, and resentment and bitterness may arise toward those perceived as receiving more love and attention. A "broken heart" may result from excessive grief or sorrow. Dysfunctions in this chakra may show themselves in relationship difficulties, which may be addictive and stifling, or alternatively superficial and transitory, with some indifference or even total withdrawal. The development of healing abilities is often associated with the opening of this chakra.

The fifth or throat chakra normally facilitates personal expression or individuality, willpower and creativity. When open, you communicate thoughts, feelings, needs, attitudes and opinions, but if this center is dysfunctional self-expression is adversely affected, creating relationship difficulties. Dishonesty and lying may occur, and other negative behavior such as fear of self-assertion, allowing yourself to become victimized by others, and gossiping may develop. Dysfunctions in this chakra may show in the voice and in use of language. If it is under-functioning, you may well have a quiet, muffled or somewhat strangled voice and tend not to speak out or up for yourself. You are likely to swallow the views and opinions of others wholesale rather than develop or express your own. If the chakra is blocked you may experience guilt and blame. If it over-functions, your voice may be loud and coarse as you impose your views on others and project on to them attributes you are unwilling to ascribe to yourself. Clairaudience and awareness of the past, present and future are associated with the opening of this chakra.

The normal functions of the sixth chakra or "third eye" are associated with clear thinking and imagery, insight and intuition. Counterclockwise movement of this chakra is associated with confused or negative ideas and images about reality. If the chakra is blocked, imagination is poor and limits creativity and problem solving. Other behavioral problems associated with blocked energy in this chakra include resistance to self-examination, suppression of intuitive capabilities, rigid thinking, obsessiveness, lack of openness to new ideas or those of others, unwillingness to learn from life experiences, and lack of self-awareness or insight. Opening of this chakra enables perception of nonphysical reality and spirit entities. Overactivity can result in feelings of possession or paranoia.

When activated, the crown chakra heightens the physical and mental senses, and promotes well-being. It provides a clear focus, and when it is open you experience a state of being that goes beyond the physical world, creating a sense of wholeness, peace, faith and a sense of purpose to life. However, when it is blocked, you become closed to spiritual experience and have little or no understanding of the spiritual experiences of others. You are likely to find life meaningless, to experience negative feelings and thoughts, to lack faith in yourself, and to fear self-development and knowledge.

Dysfunction in this chakra can be associated either with messianic inflation (believing you are a messiah) and feelings of omnipotence, or nihilism, existential depression and despair.

BECOMING ATTUNED TO SUBTLE ENERGIES

Healing with color is based upon understanding these principles. Traditionally those who did so were seers or clairvoyants, mystics who could perceive subtle energies, and thus the colors of the human energy field directly. Contemporary clairvoyants believe that others can also learn to perceive these energies. Those who cannot "see" the colors of the human energy field objectively can become attuned to vibrations of color. This sensitivity may be latent in all of us, and is reflected in commonplace descriptions of people as "in a black mood," "green with envy," "in the pink" or "blue"; and as giving out good or bad "vibes." Most people can develop heightened sensitivity to these vibrations quite easily.

Just as blindfolded subjects can distinguish colors by "feel" (see Chapter One), others can detect various physical sensations in their hands and fingertips when they pass their hands through the energy field of another person some two to three inches above the surface of the body. Heat and cold, tingling, pins and needles, pulsing, pressure or electric shock provide reliable information about pain and other symptoms of disease that can be checked by talking to the person.

THE ART OF DOWSING

An age-old technique for detecting subtle energies is dowsing. The amount and direction of the energy flowing through a chakra can be detected using a pendulum. After a few seconds the pendulum will usually begin to move. Its movement may be circular, elliptical or side to side; and smooth or erratic. The direction and radius of the movement show the amount and direction of the energy flowing through the chakra. The radius of the movement is related both to the strength and quantity of the energy flowing through the chakra and the energy of the dowser. The wider the radius the greater the energy flow. The speed of the movement indicates the rate of energy flow through the chakra. Very fast movement suggests that the chakra is being overworked, whereas a slow speed means that the energy flow through the chakra is sluggish.

Clockwise movement of the pendulum indicates an open chakra that is functioning effectively; the feelings and processes governed by it are therefore balanced and healthy. Counterclockwise movement indicates that the chakra is closed or blocked so that energy cannot flow through it. The result is that the feelings and functions governed by it are not balanced and are probably experienced negatively by the person.

Between these two extremes, various other movements may be described by the pendulum. An elliptical swing indicates a left/right imbalance of the energy flow in the body, and that one side of the body is stronger than the other. The more the circular movement of the pendulum is distorted above any given chakra the more severe is the energy distortion. A severe right/left split is suggested by a back and forth movement of the pendulum at a 45-degree angle to the vertical axis of the body; the larger the pendulum movement the greater the amount of energy contained in the distortion. Back and forth movements of the pendulum parallel to the body's vertical axis or perpendicular to it also indicate energy distortion. In the former the energy is being diverted upward and in the latter downward, suggesting that it is expressed inappropriately through a higher chakra, or suppressed. Chaotic movement means that there is considerable flux in the chakra and in its functioning. When the pendulum exhibits no movement at all the chakra is no longer functioning and is not metabolizing energy from the universal energy field. This is an unhealthy state and if maintained over time, the person will become ill.

APPLIED KINESIOLOGY

Another form of diagnosis used in healing with color is applied kinesiology. This works on a similar basis to dowsing in that it relies on imperceptible muscular responses to subtle energies to establish imbalances in the body's energy system. The healer holds a color at eye level with the left arm while extending the right arm horizontally. As each color is perceived, he or she applies gentle downward pressure to the extended right arm. Lack of resistance to this pressure suggests that the person needs the color he or she is perceiving.

SPINAL DIAGNOSIS

A more complex form of diagnosis, developed by Theo Gimbel, involves dowsing the spine with the fingers. This is based on a similar principle to radionics and involves a specimen taken from the person that is referred to as a "witness." In radionics this is usually something from the body, such as a spot of blood or lock of hair, but in Gimbel's method a signature or photograph of the subject may be used. This is placed under a chart depicting the spine. The therapist then moves the middle finger of his or her dominant hand above the chart vertebra by vertebra, feeling the sensations that arise. Vertebrae considered "inactive" produce no sensations, while active ones produce hot, cold, repelling of or tingling in the finger. This form of diagnosis is based on the idea that the subtle energy along the spinal channel is organized in sections associated with different physical and psychological functions. Each section comprises eight vertebrae, associated with colors in rainbow sequence. Diagnosis of mental and physical conditions is determined by which vertebrae — and hence which colors — are active or inactive in any section.

Gimbel's rationale is that when white light is passed through each of four carefully placed prisms, eight colored beams emerge, including magenta. He claims this is clearly visible on white paper printed with lines and bars, and results from the juxtaposition of black and white, which mixes red with ultraviolet light. The addition of this extra color produces four pairs of complementary colors when these are presented in a rainbow sequence as a color wheel. These complementary pairs are red and turquoise, orange and blue, yellow and violet, green and magenta. In combination with each other they produce white light. Gimbel stresses that complementary pairs of colors should always be used together in treatment using light in order to achieve the balance of energy essential for good health. He maintains that if a color used in treatment is not balanced by its complementary color, the condition may be made worse.

Many modern color therapists trained by Gimbel believe that there are eight colors in the spectrum and have introduced a major chakra between the throat and heart to accommodate it. In doing so they are not only departing from the traditional chakra system and practice in healing with color, but also from the accepted laws of physics.

METHODS OF HEALING WITH COLOR

COLORED LIGHT

This has been used in healing throughout history in combination with shapes, sounds, minerals, flowers, foods and other forms with the same characteristic vibrational frequency. Colored light can be projected on to various parts of the body using various devices, including lamps and filters. In many instances the light provided is defined in shapes believed to enhance the color's energetic effect.

Contemporary color therapists use full-spectrum lamps fitted with special quartz filters that can produce colors of all wavelengths and frequencies. This cannot be achieved with ordinary artificial lights because they emit some wavelengths more powerfully than others. The spectrum of light emitted from a fluorescent tube, for example, is weaker in reds than blue, green and ultraviolet.

Treatment using properly filtered full-spectrum light is powerful. Selecting the wrong color and/or exposure time may create imbalances in the body's energies; colored light should be used for healing only under the guidance of a trained practitioner. However, full-spectrum lights that produce all the wavelengths of color can be purchased and used safely and beneficially by people who spend much of their time exposed to artificial light. Indirect use of colored light may also be beneficial. In India, the traditional practice of drinking water that has been exposed to sunlight through various colored glasses is still prescribed in the treatment of specific conditions. Many color therapists use similar elixirs developed by Edwin Babbit. These preparations can be made and used at home quite safely. While use of the wrong colors will not confer any benefit on the user, they will not do any harm.

COLORED PIGMENTS

In the form of dyes and paints, colored pigments have been widely used in healing since the earliest times. These have different properties from colored light. The primary colors of pigments — red, yellow and blue — cannot be created by mixing any other colors. A mixture of these primaries looks black because together they absorb all the light that falls on them. A red pigment absorbs all the wavelengths from light except red, which it reflects; a yellow pigment absorbs everything except yellow; and a blue pigment absorbs everything but blue. When a pair of pigment primaries are mixed together they produce secondaries; red and yellow make orange, red and blue make violet, and yellow and blue make green, producing the seven principal colors traditionally associated with the color spectrum.

The general principles followed by color therapists are that energies can be stimulated by encouraging everyday exposure to certain colors. This can be done through clothes and accessories or in the decoration and furnishing of your living and working environments, and by eating certain foods. The principle of resonance is used to determine which energies are expressed most by an individual. A person who usually wears a lot of red is assumed to be resonating with that vibration, and so may benefit from adding other colors, notably the "cooler" calming shades of green and blue, if she tends to become "overheated" or overexcited or suffer from ailments associated with an excess of red energy. By contrast, someone who suffers from not having enough of this energy and avoids wearing the color may benefit from wearing it and from being in red surroundings. Such a person may also benefit from eating red meat, and food such as beets, radishes, tomatoes, red-skinned fruits and spices such as cayenne, cloves and capsicum pepper. These should be avoided by those with an excess of red energy.

This awareness forms the basis of Ayurveda, the traditional medicine of India and one of the oldest systems of healing in the world. Similar principles are also fundamental to traditional Chinese medicine.

GEMSTONES AND CRYSTALS

These are widely used to augment color on and around the body and may be worn as talismans, amulets and jewelry, placed over the chakras or in the energy field of the body. In treatment, they are used with minerals and metals. Gemstones and crystals ground or powdered into water have for many many years been prescribed as oral medication in the Ayurveda tradition. However, it has long been understood that the healing properties of gems are transferred to water or another liquid in which the stone is immersed, and gem elixirs have been used in healing since ancient times. They are prepared by potentizing water containing gemstones through exposure to natural light, and then taken by mouth. When applied externally they can be combined with creams and essential oils to be used in massage and added to baths. Gems may also be placed in baths with the appropriate elixir.

ESSENTIAL OILS

Derived from flowering plants to augment the effects of color in healing, the use of essential oils is also an ancient practice. Today an increasing number of people combine color and aromatherapy in healing.

Color is often the link between essential oils and the chakras. Patricia Davis identifies essential oils traditionally classed as Base Notes in perfumery and reddish in color as resonating with the base chakra. Hence myrrh may have an energizing effect when base chakra energy is low. Davis suggests that bergamot and inula, both green oils, connect with the heart chakra. With melissa, an oil with a "green" aroma, bergamot and inula may be valuable where there is an energy blockage between the second and third chakras.

Two oils are identified by Davis as particularly appropriate to the throat chakra, German blue chamomile and the paler blue English chamomile; juniper has indigo berries that correspond with the brow chakra; lavender works with the crown chakra. These oils may be applied by way of massage, baths, inhalers or burners, or simply by putting a couple of drops on handkerchiefs, pillows and the like.

Inger Naess of Norway has developed a line of color oils for use in baths under the tradename Color Bath. These are pure essential oils used to balance chakra energies. They can be used to increase or reduce certain energies: a person with a lot of red energy should tone down this energy by taking a green bath, whereas someone needing red energy should take a red bath.

FLOWER ESSENCES

Gem elixirs are often used along with flower essences — they are believed to have a synergistic effect. The flower essences are produced in much the same way as elixirs — by potentizing water containing flowers in full sunlight — and used in similar ways.

The color of the plant from which the essences are derived is perhaps less important than the "color" associated with its vibration.

Edward Bach, the physician who was the first person in modern times to develop a system of healing with flower essences, organized his flower remedies into seven groups, each associated with a different color and shown on a color wheel chart still produced by the Bach Center in England. The energy imbalances treated by the remedies in each of these groups broadly correspond with the function of the chakras. Although Bach made no reference to chakras or color in developing his system, it is nevertheless probable that color is a reliable guide to their selection and use.

PSYCHOLOGICAL METHODS OF HEALING WITH COLOR

The methods of diagnosis and treatment described above basically rely on physical sensitivity. However, traditional methods of diagnosis and treatment depend more on psychological sensitivity, and therefore on intuition and insight — literally inner sensing or seeing. The ancients recognized that mental images are energy forms with numerous applications in healing, and may involve any of the senses or a combination of them. It is not the case, as is often assumed, that images are necessarily visual. An image involves not merely "seeing" a picture in the mind's eye but sensing or experiencing it in various ways. As Barbara Ann Brennan writes, "Perceiving means receiving. Perception is receiving what is already there."

Much of what "is there" in life, though, is difficult to grasp because it cannot easily be conceived or conveyed verbally. Images allow many nonverbal phenomena such as physical, emotional and spiritual experiences to be represented in the mind. They therefore provide a way of thinking about what was formerly "unthinkable." As such, they facilitate conscious awareness of much that is ordinarily unconscious, and so they can be used not only to develop awareness of the effects of subtle energies and color, but also to provide reliable information about these phenomena. Buddhist traditions emphasize the importance of identifying with the chakras by focusing awareness on them and thus sensing rather than thinking about them. Color images produced in this way are used diagnostically in various approaches to healing with color. (See Part Two.)

VISUALIZATION

Forming images in the mind's eye, or visualization, is widely used in healing with color. As Brennan points out, this has an entirely different function:

The process of visualization is actively creating. In visualization you create a picture in your mind and give it energy. If you continue to hold it clearly in your mind and give it energy, you can eventually create it in your life. You have thus given it form and substance. The clearer the image and the more emotional energy you project into it, the more you will be able to create it in your life.

Contemporary research on imagery lends support to this view. Much has been written over the past twenty years which confirms that images are indeed a powerful force, and can have profound physical and psychological effects. According to Dr. Larry Dossey, these effects are as potent as those produced by any drug; imagery should be regarded as medicine in the truest sense of the word.

It is now known that imagining something is essentially the same as perceiving it in the external world. Simply imagining sucking a lemon, for example, has a direct effect on the salivary glands. The effects of imagery on heart rate, blood pressure, blood flow, electrodermal activity and immune response have all been confirmed in experiments.

This principle underpins various practices used in healing with color, notably color visualization and meditating on colored images. By imagining color you produce vibrations of a certain frequency, which, when directed to the energy centers of the body, can produce various psychological and physical effects. Visualization of and meditation on color are also thought to strengthen its energies and increase its healing properties. Meditation on colored light, pigment, crystals, gemstones, minerals, elixirs, flowers and foods used in healing is believed to reinforce their effects. In traditional Indian and Chinese medicine, visualizing light being drawn into the body in various ways is recommended for self-healing.

Visualization of light and color also plays a large part in Tibetan medicine. Brilliant white or colored light is imagined radiating from a deity and flowing through your being, purifying it mentally and physically. This light can be directed by you to a diseased area of the body, or outward into the universe to heal others. In Chinese medicine, people are encouraged to enhance, redirect and normalize vital energies by imagining them in various ways. A common breathing exercise is to imagine breathing in colored light. This is also practiced in many other traditions, ancient and modern, together with other kinds of color imagery.

The practice of channelling or sending color to vitalize someone else's depleted energies is common in healing with color.

This involves visualizing a color and imagining "sending" it to the person to be treated. In this way color may be channelled through the hands directly into the body of a person, or it may be sent to a person at some distance through the universal energy field.

Healers often use colored crystals as wands to direct subtle energy into the chakras, and at Hygeia Studios, England, a hand-held torch that focuses light through a stained-glass filter and a clear quartz crystal has been developed for the same purpose.

Images can thus be used both in sensing and sending energies, and these functions are combined in many different ancient and modern approaches to healing with color. These two processes are fundamental to Therapeutic Touch, developed by Dolores Krieger, former Professor of Nursing at New York University. Therapeutic Touch is now regarded here and in Canada as a natural extension of professional nursing skills.

Training in Therapeutic Touch takes place in five stages. First, the healer must learn to relax and focus her attention inward in order to achieve a meditative state. Next, she makes an assessment of the patient's energies by passing her hands through the energy field surrounding the body some two to three inches above its surface.

Differences in energy flow resulting from imbalance are detected through sensations in the healer's hands, such as variations in temperature, pins and needles, tingling, pulsing, pressure or electric shock and associated color imagery. The healer then relieves congestion by employing stroking or sweeping gestures away from the affected part, and after washing or shaking her hands to remove the charge picked up from the patient, places her hands on either side of the affected area and imagines directing energy into it. The energy is modulated through use of color imagery so the healer mentally pictures sending blue energy to cool or sedate, red to warm or stimulate, yellow to energize, and continues to do so until the patient's body feels balanced.

In Part Two you are invited to combine these techniques of sensing and sending color energy by way of imagery, and thereby discover and develop your true colors as a means for healing yourself and others.

PART TWO

—

DISCOVERING
YOUR TRUE COLORS

3

Emory

DEVELOPING COLOR CONSCIOUSNESS

Implicit in healing with color is the ideal of perfect health as symbolized by a rainbow. Like a rainbow, a healthy person should distribute all energies, wavelengths and colors in a balanced way. The aim of healing with color is to attune people to their rainbow, to vitalize the chakras and exhort them to a healthy level. It is therefore concerned with increasing awareness of color, its subtle effects and influences on life, and with the development of what might be called color consciousness.

The first step in developing color consciousness is to identify the colors that figure in your life and the experiences you associate with them. You can begin by answering the following questions:

- What colors are you wearing now?

- Why did you choose to wear these clothes?

- How do you feel when wearing them?

- How do these colors compare with those you normally wear?

- What is your favorite color?

- What is your least favorite color?

- When you look into your wardrobe, what colors do you see?

- Does any one color or colors predominate?

- What colors are missing or not well represented there?

- What color or colors would you never wear and why?

- Are there any colors that you would like to wear but cannot or do not wear? What are your reasons for not doing so?

- How frequently do you not find anything to wear that you feel comfortable in?

- What colors predominate in your main living areas?

- What colors predominate in your work space?

- What color is your bedroom?

- What color is your car and its interior upholstery?

The significance of your answers lies in the fact that a person's energies express themselves through color. The principle underlying this idea is that of resonance. Energies that naturally vibrate at certain frequencies are excited by energies in the environment vibrating at precisely the same frequency. These energies "strike a chord," quite literally. If you pluck the E string of a violin, for example, the E string of a nearby violin will begin to vibrate in harmony because both strings are tuned and responsive to a particular frequency.

In the same way, certain colors strike a chord with us when their vibrations match our own. We are likely to prefer these to colors whose vibrations we do not resonate with, just as we tend to like people we consider to be on the same wavelength as ourselves and to dislike those with whom we don't get along. Our dislike of certain colors suggests that we are not resonating with them, and thus not functioning effectively in respect to these frequencies. So color preference is an indication of the subtle energies we are attuned to.

Even though we express liking certain colors, we may avoid them. How often have you heard someone say that she likes a color but doesn't wear it or live with it because it is "too much" or "a little over the top"? This suggests that she doesn't want to excite these particular frequencies, maybe because she is overenergized in that area, probably because it is compensating for energies that are not being properly used elsewhere. So when a color is avoided, either because these energies are not being used or because they are being overused, the color preference shows the need to balance these energies.

The quantity of energy used by a person is as important as its quality, and some idea of this can be gained from the intensity of color preferred. Many women express a preference for pastel or diluted shades and tend to tone down bright or strong colors. Some of those who like bright colors don't wear them because they don't want to draw attention to themselves. By doing so, they are reflecting social conventions regarding the expression of gender-appropriate energies. Can it be coincidental that the color pink, traditionally associated with women in Western culture, has calming effects and suppresses the expression of anger and aggression? Or that blue, traditionally associated with baby boys in our culture, is the color of self-expression? Women often choose to wear navy blue to work, and especially for job interviews and business meetings with men, again most likely because this color has a subduing effect and expresses control.

Perhaps even more alarming is the number of women who avoid wearing colors they like because they have been told by others that the colors don't suit them. These may be color counselors who base their judgments on hair or eye color and skin tone rather than on the balanced expression of personal energies. Once again this highlights the impact of social constraints on self-expression. Men, however, often express a preference for shades of blue, which is consistent with social conditioning and expectations. Many men also wear muddy colors that women often describe as "mucky." Khaki colors may not so much camouflage the individual but show clearly that hearty green energies are dysfunctional, just as earthy shades may suggest that basic physical and creative energies are not being properly expressed. Men in grey have almost become an emblem of our times — both a depressing thought and a depressing color.

Many women state emphatically that they would never wear yellow or orange, colors associated with intellect, willpower and strong passions, again reflecting stereotypical views on the energies women in our culture should suppress. Although there may be fewer strictures about men appearing "bright" and energetic, they tend not to wear these clothes in the workplace and confine them to leisure wear or to ties. Purple is avoided equally by men and women, suggesting the lack of a spiritual dimension in their lives.

Generally, few people wear or even possess a full range of colored clothes. The garments they wear tend to reflect one end or the other of the color spectrum, or its mid-range. Some possess clothes of all but one color. A small minority of people wear only one color. Even those who possess a wide range of colors may wear some of these more than others. This may reflect other social conventions such as fashion, or more idiosyncratic factors like physical state and mood.

If you find that you wear only a limited range of colors, identify those you rarely or never wear, and consult the details in Chapter Two about the appropriate chakra. Remember that red is associated with the base chakra, orange with the second chakra, yellow with the third chakra, green with the fourth, blue with the fifth, dark blue or indigo with the sixth, and purple or violet with the crown chakra. In this way you should be able to identify the energies these colors relate to, and their implications for your psychological and physical well-being.

A COLOR DIARY

You can develop awareness of the effects of color on your physical state, moods, feelings, attitudes, interests, activities and relationships by keeping a color diary. Try this first for one week. Every day record what colors and color combinations you wear while doing various things, and note how you feel physically, mentally, emotionally and spiritually as you do so. This sounds easier than it is. You may change your clothes several times a day, usually without thinking about it. Keeping a diary of this kind requires you to become aware of those changes, when and where they occur, and their effects on a number of different personal levels.

You may find that the colors lacking in your clothes are also absent from your living and working environment, or that you wear certain colors to compensate for lack of color in these settings. Try keeping a diary for a second week, adding your feelings about your usual surroundings and your reactions to decor, lighting and such.

You may identify with Jackie, who was initially delighted to be able to save money on the furnishings of her new house, which was decorated and carpeted throughout in shades of grey. After four weeks she found that she couldn't stay in the house for any length of time without becoming depressed, and when her husband commented that she always seemed to be going out she insisted that they redecorate despite the cost. Jackie decorated the living room in shades of pink and green which she, her family and friends found very relaxing. She also painted her older daughter's bedroom pink, but in an attempt to brighten the bedroom of her three-year-old daughter, painted it bright yellow. Some time later she realized that the child had never slept through the night in this room, whereas she would sleep throughout the night in her sister's room.

Maria changed the feminine pink shades of her bedroom when she married and her husband moved into her house. She subsequently attributed the cooling and eventual breakdown of their relationship to the blue/grey shades she chose instead.

Graham, who felt "chilled out" by the pale blue decor of his friend's living room, insisted on changing the blues chosen as bedroom decoration by his wife to pink, which he felt was warmer and softer. Jim, a physical education teacher, found his school's grey sports hall totally depressing, an observation shared by other teachers obliged to proctor examinations in there. The school inspectors agreed and suggested that a brighter color might improve both athletic and scholastic performance.

By contrast, the managers of a company whose workers tended to congregate and chat in the men's restroom solved the problem by painting the walls bright orange. As a result it was no longer a "rest room," and the workers hastily returned to their work. Carl, the director of an art gallery, was puzzled as to why an interactive multimedia exhibition designed for three- to five-year-olds failed to excite them. His staff, who had anticipated having to deal with chaos caused by up to sixty children playing with spectacular computer-generated games, were astonished to find that the children instead seemed restrained and somber. No one at the gallery had given much thought to the overall color and lighting of the display. The walls, furniture and furnishings were predominantly dark blue, lit by subdued fluorescent lighting which is low in red, orange and yellow wavelengths, and distorts colors, making them seem more blue. This created a subdued environment almost totally lacking in the reds, oranges and yellows needed to stimulate and excite children of this age.

By keeping a detailed diary you may be able to identify those colors that resonate with and are comfortable for you. You may then wish to experiment with colors you don't normally wear or expose yourself to. Pam found that when wearing brown, a color she often wore teamed with fashionable creams, taupes and beige, she tended to withdraw mentally and emotionally. By experimenting as suggested, first with turquoise earrings and necklaces, then with scarves and eventually with sweaters and dresses, she found that she could speak up for herself more and that her normally hushed voice gained timbre. As a result of being more confident about expressing herself Pam went on to try purples, violets, magenta and pinks and was astonished not only to feel more vibrant but also to find others telling her she looked years younger.

Similarly, Ann, who hadn't worn green in years, began to experiment with it, initially by walking in the countryside and then by wearing a green scarf. She soon found that she was emotionally calmer and more relaxed. As she brought more and more green into her life she realized that she had healed a heart "broken" some years before by the death of a loved one.

Experimenting with color and observing its effects is not a matter of thinking of color, but experiencing it. As Barbara Ann Brennan points out, in energetic terms thought is a yellow vibration, so irrespective of what color you think of, you will create yellow. So you need to experiment with what it is like to "be" in a state of blue. This involves being aware of how you feel when you wear blue or sit in a blue light, and of what blue means to you — how it looks, feels and sounds. In order to develop color consciousness you need to explore your relationship to every color in this way. The exercises in the chapters that follow will help you do this.

4

RELAXING WITH COLOR

If asked "How do you relax?" what would your response be? Would you say you watch TV, read books, complete crossword puzzles, go for walks, engage in sports or have a few drinks with friends? Whatever your answer, you are unlikely to say that you "cease to maintain the tension in the muscles of your body." Yet this is precisely how we relax. Generally, when people think they are relaxed they are not. They may remain mentally active, physically aroused, anxious, fidgety, restless and react to the slightest noise. Their blood pressure may be raised and their pulse rate increased. They may breathe irregularly, swallow frequently, or show involuntary reflexes such as wrinkling the forehead and stiffness in the muscles of the face, all of which indicate residual tension.

In true relaxation, tension is absent, breathing is regular, there is no reflex swallowing, pulse rate and blood pressure decrease, and you sit or lie quietly with flaccid limbs and motionless eyelids. Less obviously but more importantly, the mental processes that generate bodily tension in the first place are switched off — the habitual thoughts, concerns, preoccupations and anxieties. The mind is therefore blank in the sense that the "sound" has been turned down, but it is not empty. Images present themselves fleetingly. Just as television transforms electromagnetic energies into sights and sounds, your mind transforms subtle energies into various sensory images. It is no more true to say that these images are produced because the sound is off than it is to say that turning the sound down produces pictures on a television screen. They have been there all along but have been unattended to. Similarly, many people "watch" TV mainly by listening to the soundtrack and pay little attention to the images on the screen. When the sound is turned down they are obliged to look at these images to find out what is going on.

In much the same way, most people need to turn down the sound — the chatter of verbal thought which acts as a constant soundtrack accompanying everything that goes on in and around them — before they can receive the images produced by their own mind. This occurs spontaneously during sleep and at other times when the mind wanders from its usual preoccupations. However, although dreams, daydreams and fantasies can provide a great deal of information about the self, they tend to be dismissed as fanciful. Relaxation enables us to focus attention on the images we receive so we can understand their meaning and the information they convey about aspects of ourselves of which we are ordinarily unaware.

If you have begun to notice some of the effects of color in your life you may want to develop your awareness further. The following exercise, which combines relaxation and imagery, will help you to do this. It can be repeated as often as you like because it reflects the energies that are being

expressed at any time and will change as you and the cir-
cumstances of your life alter (although certain features may
remain constant). Awareness of both variable and constant
features will give you greater insight into how effectively
you are using your energies, enabling you to monitor and
balance them. I recommend that you take your time and
allow twenty minutes for the exercise. It is a good idea to
record the instructions on cassette or to ask someone to read
them to you until you are familiar enough with the steps to
do without such help.

EXERCISE 1
SEEING YOUR TRUE COLORS

Find somewhere quiet and make yourself comfortable,
either sitting or lying (preferably the former so you don't go
to sleep).

Having done this, become aware of your surroundings and
how you feel. Then close your eyes (if this is not possible
because of any physical problems, or difficult because of
contact lenses, focus on a fixed point or object within your
line of vision, such as a mark on a wall, ceiling or floor).

Now gradually withdraw your attention from your surroundings, and bring it to the boundary between your body
and adjacent surfaces. As you do so, notice whether the contact is uncomfortable or painful, and adjust your position to
make yourself as comfortable as possible. You may find that
you need to remove restrictive clothing, shoes, jewelry or
glasses. At any point in the exercise when you feel the need
to, adjust your position to reduce pain or discomfort.

When you are positioned comfortably, turn your attention to
your feelings. How *do* you feel? Do you feel silly or guilty
about taking time to do the exercise, reluctant or impatient
to get on with it?

How self-conscious are you? Are you worried about being
seen by others, or that they are nearby? Are you worried

that you might not be able to "do" the exercise, or what you might discover about yourself if you can? Your reactions may reflect some of the basic anxieties of your life. If during any part of the exercise thoughts, feelings, memories or impressions come to mind, make a mental note of them since they may be significant.

Now bring your attention to your toes and tighten them as much as you can. Keep doing this until you can identify the extent of its effects throughout your body and then let go, observing as you do so the difference between the sensations of tightening and letting go. Pause for a moment as you focus awareness on your toes before repeating this action two or three times. Then, progressing slowly upward from your toes, repeat this process, tightening and letting go in turn your legs, knees, thighs, buttocks, lower back, stomach, chest, shoulders, both arms and hands, your neck, brow, eyes, nose, lips, mouth and jaw.

Then bring your attention back to your toes, and starting with them tighten successively all the other parts of your body so that it is tense throughout its length. Increase this tightness as much as you can, and hold it for several moments before letting go. Allow the resulting sensation of floppiness to spread throughout your body. Then repeat this action twice more. Your body should now be fully relaxed, with your jaw slack and your mouth open. If they are not fully relaxed, repeat the action, accentuating the tightness in your jaw and letting your mouth fall open when you relax.

Having done so, breathe in through your nose and out through your open mouth, observing how this feels and its effects on your body. Still breathing in this way, spend a few moments becoming aware of the sensations throughout your body. If relaxed, your limbs and body should feel heavy and warm. Scan your body from top to bottom, noting any tightness, discomfort or pain that persists despite these attempts.

Now focus your attention on your chest and observe your breathing. Is it regular or irregular; shallow or deep; difficult or easy?

Still focusing on your chest, imagine that there is a butterfly resting there and that as you breathe in and out it gradually spreads its wings to their full extent as though you are breathing energy and life into it. Look at it carefully, noting its size and color and your feelings toward it. When the butterfly's wings are fully extended and it seems prepared to fly off, breathe out deeply and watch it fly away. Be aware of your thoughts and feelings as it does so. Then imagine that you follow it, noting all the sensations you experience.

After a while it comes to a rest, and as you do likewise, you find yourself in a pleasant situation where you feel relaxed, comfortable and secure. Every detail of this place becomes vivid as you pay careful attention to the sights, sounds, smells and sensations there. When you realize that you can be really yourself there, begin to pay particular attention to color and allow yourself to experience it fully. As you do so, take note of how you feel and any features of the "real" you that seem particularly significant.

Don't try to direct your thoughts to create specific images, and don't censor them. Simply allow images to emerge spontaneously — receive them as they arise. Also be aware of any difficulty you have in imagining yourself in such a place, and of any distracting thoughts, feelings, memories or sensations that arise. Don't dwell on these, but don't try to suppress them. Merely make a mental note and allow them to disappear.

Having entered into this experience as fully as you can, ask yourself what its significance might be and what the different colors you have seen may represent. When you have answered these questions as best you can, allow the image to fade and return to ordinary awareness by opening your eyes.

Try recording your experience on cassette or in a written log so that you can reflect upon it and refer to it later. Doing so will help you to cross-reference and interrelate it with experiences from later exercises. The following commentary may also help you to understand the personal significance of your imagery more fully. If you feel you may be influenced by knowing others' responses, don't read the commentary until you have completed and recorded the exercise.

COMMENTARY

The butterfly image used in the above exercise is a very potent symbol of the self. The ancient Greeks used the term *psyche* to refer to both the butterfly and the self or soul — the spiritual nature of the individual. Universally, the butterfly represents spiritual qualities, transformation, metamorphosis, change and freedom. Paying attention to this image invariably reveals important personal issues.

From the responses of large numbers of people, it seems clear that the colors of the butterfly reflect the energies that they are expressing currently, whereas the colors of the place the butterfly leads them to represent the energies they need to express in order to really be themselves. The image focuses awareness on personal authenticity; that is, on how much of the true self is suppressed in order to conform with social pressures and expectations — and what might be expressed if the person were to show their true colors.

Butterflies naturally occur in all colors and color combinations, but this is not reflected in response to the above exercise. Typically, solid red, orange, brown or pink butterflies don't appear, whereas those that are completely yellow, green, blue, turquoise, purple and white are often described. All-black butterflies are described only rarely, and completely brown butterflies are very uncommon. White reflects all colors and suggests healthy functioning, where all energies are being used and expressed in a balanced way.

The deeper the color imagined the more intensely the color energies represented by the butterfly are being expressed at the present time. When the color is bright this energy may predominate over all other energies and need balancing accordingly. Bright yellow butterflies may therefore be imagined by headstrong people who intellectualize everything and whose mental attitude colors everything including sex, feelings and self-expression. Such rational people speak from the head rather than the heart, and may be quite out of touch with their feelings. Typically, one woman who imagined a huge bright yellow butterfly reported feeling envious because she couldn't identify with it.

People who imagine bright green butterflies may allow their emotions to color everything, whereas those who imagine blue butterflies may be rather selfish, seeing everything in terms of how it affects and reflects on themselves. Bright purple butterflies often indicate individuals whose spiritual concerns predominate, sometimes with the result that they are out of touch with ordinary reality.

Dilute colors appear to be associated with energies and potential not being adequately used or expressed. In some cases this is extreme. Transparent butterflies suggest no sense of presence. One woman who imagined a very pale butterfly saw this as accurately reflecting the fact that she did not express anything of her true self.

Usually, however, color is evident, but pale. Pale yellow, green and blue butterflies are often imagined. Sometimes these colors are described as washed out, which suggests that this energy has been drained. In relation to green energies, this shows that the emotional energies have been overworked, which has implications for immune functioning. (The relationship between emotional trauma and immune-related diseases such as cancers is in fact well established.)

"Drained" yellow energies suggest that intellectual and work-related demands may be taking their toll, and that the person is susceptible to stress and related physical and psychological problems. Washed out blue energies are likely to indicate poor self-expression and a tendency to throat and speech disorders.

When white butterflies are tinged with other colors, fringed or tipped with color or have spots or patches of color, this suggests that these energies are somewhat out of balance, to the extent indicated by the intensity of the colors. A woman who imagined a white butterfly with pale yellow spots had little confidence in her intellectual ability, and didn't express her views in case she revealed her shortcomings.

Orange and white butterflies are quite often imagined, and indicate that physical energies need regulating. Pale orange suggests that the person is lacking in energy and vitality. Bright orange, on the other hand, tends to characterize people who are highly energetic and constantly on the go, such as Jan, whose excessive energy was represented in numerous vivid orange spots on an otherwise white butterfly, shown in her hyperactivity and inability to relax.

The size of the butterfly appears to reflect the potential energy available to the individual. Its behavior and the person's attitudes toward it are also significant. Large butterflies suggest considerable potential, which is, however, often underused. People may attempt to restrain the butterfly because they fear losing it, and flatten it in the attempt. One man reported holding his butterfly "close to his chest" so that its true colors couldn't be seen. Many butterflies are extremely delicate and fragile. Some flutter their wings but are unable to stretch them fully or fly. Some crumple horribly at the first attempt, while others remain with wings outstretched but are still unable to fly. Others flutter their wings and make gestures toward flying without actually doing so.

A number of butterflies are imagined as tattoos, silhouettes, templates, appliqué decorations, origami or cardboard cutouts. So although they may be colorful, they are not alive.

These images indicate the extent to which individuals may stifle or restrict expression of their potential, or crumple in the face of their own reality.

Whatever their shape or substance, butterflies usually combine several colors. Where one color is tinged with black this suggests that a trace of negativity runs throughout the expression of this energy and that it is not being fully realized. Wings that are black tipped or fringed may indicate that negativity interferes with the full expression of these energies. Red fringed with black is suggestive of insecurity and poor self-confidence, especially in relation to the body and sexuality. Orange tipped with black is suggestive of negative reactions, the tendency to doubt your gut feelings, and feelings of powerlessness.

Yellow tipped with black may suggest negative thoughts and attitudes, and green tipped with black may signify emotions such as resentment and jealousy, and difficulties in relationships. Blue tipped with black may indicate coolness, distance and aloofness, while purple tipped with black may be associated with feelings of dread, despair, hopelessness and lack of purpose.

Black spots, splashes, blobs or patches suggest negativity or a more intermittent failure fully to express energies. These may be thought of as blemishes on the individual's character — not in a critical way, but inasmuch as they represent potential whose expression is patchy in quality, occurrence and intensity.

One woman, who imagined a large, deep green, exotic butterfly whose secondary wings were banded and barred with black, saw this as reflecting very strong emotions that were sometimes not fully or appropriately expressed. Indeed she felt so strongly about some issues that she couldn't allow herself to acknowledge fully, much less express, these feelings.

A person's imagery may combine several of the above features. One woman was alarmed by the size of her imagined butterfly, which spread very wide across her chest. Every time it attempted to fly off she tried to catch it until finally it crumpled completely. Afterward she acknowledged always having had difficulty holding onto anything in life, and losing what she wanted by trying too hard. She recognized that the color of her butterfly — pale mauve edged with black — was significant, as was the fact that she was dressed in the same color. The woman associated purple with mourning and with the sadness of being a loser; she realized that mauve, a diluted purple, represented her attempt to conceal this sadness from others so as to be acceptable to them. Only the black edges of the butterfly's wings revealed her true feelings.

This woman interpreted the significance of the colors in her imagery having had no prior knowledge or understanding of their traditional meanings. From the traditional perspective, purple is associated with spiritual issues such as purpose in life, with transcendence, joy and ecstatic experience.

The butterflies imagined by many people combine several colors. Some liken theirs to a Red Admiral, a common butterfly that is predominantly red, orange and brown with some areas of black. Its colors are associated with the lower chakra energies and functions. Where brown appears in imagery it indicates stagnant energy. Muddy reds may suggest lack of sexual fulfillment or creativity, and brown juxtaposed with red, suggests that expression of this basic energy alternates — sometimes quite intense, at other times blocked. In conjunction with orange it suggests lack of emotional vitality, sluggishness and feelings of powerlessness.

Deborah hadn't seen much significance in her Red Admiral until she related its colors to these features. She then admitted to deep-seated insecurities and a lack of confidence that had resulted in emotional difficulties and body image problems. By her thirties, having been both anorexic and bulimic, she had become obese, and she admitted to wearing dark colors to hide her weight. Deborah also had difficulty expressing herself, and as a result she had fared badly at interviews and was unfulfilled in her job.

Following the exercise, where she imagined following the Red Admiral to a tropical paradise of blue skies, lush green vegetation and vivid red, orange and yellow flowers, she decided to wear these colors. Deborah was subsequently delighted not only to find her confidence greatly increased but also, following an interview, to be offered a job in which she felt she could show her true colors.

As Deborah's imagery reveals, clues are provided by the situation the butterfly leads to, showing how the energies can be balanced. One woman identified strongly with the huge, turquoise-blue butterfly she imagined. Like her, it was a high flyer, and she was initially happy to follow it up into the sky; but the higher it flew, the more uncomfortable she became. She began to feel vulnerable and concerned that the butterfly would be "shot down." She felt that to go higher would not be "right" for her and was therefore greatly relieved when suddenly it led her to an Amazon rainforest that was predominantly bright green but full of flowers of all colors. She took this as a sign of the anxiety she felt as a high-flying professional without any real sense of direction in her life.

Taken together, the butterfly and the place it leads you to present a full spectrum of colors, which represent everyone's true colors and the healthy expression of their full range of energies or potential.

5

IDENTIFYING ENERGY BLOCKS THROUGH COLOR

———

Tension is blocked energy — energy trapped in muscles and unable to flow. Nevertheless, tension involves considerable energy, which is why when you are tense you feel tired and drained. Lying in bed with tense muscles may be a greater drain on your energy than digging in the garden all day. This is because physical work, after an initial effort, is reduced in inertia, whereas tightening muscles and sustaining this tension requires constant energy. So paradoxically, hard work may involve less "work" than so-called rest. Maintaining muscular tension over time uses considerable energy, is progressively tiring, and imposes strain on your body. If you expend too much energy, your body becomes worn out doing nothing due to excessive use of adenosine triphosphate or cyclic TCP, the basic chemical used in nerve and muscle cells.

People with chronic tension often become locked into a self-perpetuating cycle where, although tired, their muscular tensions prevent them from relaxing or sleeping, further exhausting them so that any action requires more effort. The fundamental problem for such people is that generally they are unaware that they are tense, and because they don't realize that they are creating tension, they don't know how they are doing it or what they can do to stop it. They are also unaware of the energies tied up in maintaining this tension, and its implications for their health, well-being and effective functioning. The following exercise uses color imagery to help you to assess whether or not you are using your energies effectively.

Exercise 2

Find somewhere to sit or lie comfortably with your eyes closed or focused on a fixed point.

Imagine you are lying under a pleasantly warm sun and that you can feel its rays warming but not burning your skin. Imagine that the warmth is penetrating your skin and soothing your aches and pains. As you scan your body slowly from the toes upward, you can feel the warmth dissolving the tension, which is pictured in the form of ice. The ice becomes drops of warm fluid that flow in streams through your body and seep out into the ground through the pores of your skin, leaving your body feeling heavy and warm. Notice any areas where the ice seems particularly dense or resistant to the sun's warmth, focusing your attention on each of these until the ice has dissolved away.

Continue to scan upward through your body until all your tensions have dissolved. Having done so, now focus your attention on your head. Imagine the sun's rays are penetrating your mind, gently dissolving your anxieties, conflicts, confusions, concerns and preoccupations. Allow these to seep away, leaving your mind and body a clear channel without obstruction. Then pay attention to the tensions that have flowed out of you. Imagine that they form an expanse of water. Observe it carefully, noting its significant features and paying particular attention to its color, clarity, depth and movement. When you are picturing it as vividly as you can, ask yourself the following questions:

1) What might this image tell me about my energies and how effectively I am using them?

2) What can I learn from it?

When you have answered the questions, gradually allow the image to fade, open your eyes and return to ordinary consciousness. Then record or write your experience down, noting the location and nature of your "energy blocks," the manner in which they dissolved, and how easy or difficult it was to dissolve them. Also note details of the water imagery, paying particular attention to the features of color, clarity, depth and movement, concluding with an assessment of what these features might indicate about your energies and how effectively you are using them.

The following commentary, drawn from observations made by people who have undertaken this exercise, might help you to understand your own imagery.

COMMENTARY

The expanse of water imagined in the above exercise is formed from dissolving tension. It will therefore tend to reflect the predominant areas of tension within your body and the energies that are bound up there. Given this, it is not surprising that some people describe the water they imagine as red, although red is not a color usually associated with water. Indeed it often strikes people as odd or puzzling if they are not familiar with the esoteric concepts of subtle energies, chakras and the aura.

The water may be imagined as reflecting the colors of the setting sun — orange or yellow. Just as the colors of the setting sun bring an end to the vitalizing rays of the day and onset of night, so too when imagined they suggest that the person's vital physical and mental energies are subdued and on the wane.

Green water often impresses us as cold in appearance and unwelcoming. When imagined in this exercise it suggests lack of emotional warmth resulting from blocked heart energies. Blue water suggests that self-expression is ordinarily blocked, and the darker the blue the more likely it is that the person also lacks self-insight.

Purple water may embody the reflections of mountains, its depths representing an inversion of a person's highest aspiration.

Brown water is often imagined. One man who did so could find no significance in this until he was asked how water becomes brown. John replied by saying that it contained material in suspension such as effluent or sewage, and this corresponded with his experience of himself as "full of shit."

Grey water can have a similar significance. Sheila imagined cloudy grey water in which people had washed their dirty clothes, promptly triggering an association with the phrase "washing dirty linen in public." She subsequently recognized that this resulted from becoming involved in other people's unpleasant business and allowing her thinking to become clouded by it.

A black oily or greasy "film" is sometimes described on the surface of the water, which suggests something having been "dumped" or imposed on it from elsewhere. This "pollution" reflects the negativity that often accompanies a person's acting in accordance with the wishes of others rather than expressing oneself.

Black water, having absorbed all the possible colors expressed from the body, indicates profound negativity and tension amounting to rigidity and torpor. Black is associated with lack of clarity and vision.

Color and clarity are often closely connected. The degree of clarity may be an indication of the self-insight a person has.

Unclear areas may indicate unexplored or unacknowledged aspects of the self, fears, anxieties and other features that people don't wish to look into too closely — their darker aspects — and tend to avoid.

Some people report being unable to see into this water because of reflections. This suggests that their reflection of other things or people — such as social expectations — prevents them from seeing their own depths and potential, which as a result are uncharted and unused. Many people's energies are taken up in creating or living up to the images expected by others.

Some people cannot easily determine the extent or depth of the water they imagine. Such people have difficulty in perceiving their own potential. Some people are aware that the water they imagine is part of a bigger expanse of water and that they have far greater potential than they are using. Others are aware of drawing on inexhaustible sources, while some see their sources as limited to a puddle or trickle. Attention to the clarity of water tends to highlight features of depth and limits or boundaries.

Other people recognize that their surface features give a false impression of what is going on below. In some cases the surface of the water may be calm and belie a churning underneath, or the surface may be agitated and wild, but tranquil below. The surface colors may also differ from those beneath. These features suggest the ways in which some people consciously or unwittingly conceal themselves and their true colors, and the difference between their inner and outer selves.

For most people the movement of the water they imagine is striking and significant. It may be sluggish or slow, suggesting insufficient energy; or rushing, frenzied and in some cases dangerously out of control. Dissipation of energy is a common feature of the imagery.

Michael interpreted his dry river in a chalk landscape as reflecting his need to withdraw into himself occasionally to restore his energy. Pamela realized that the waves she saw bobbing up and down on the surface of the water corresponded to her mood cycles. She felt okay when she was "on the up" and her "head was above water," but frightened when she was overwhelmed or "down."

The movement of the water is usually determined to some extent by the nature of the restrictions on it. Whereas some people imagine the water as expansive, others see it as very confined: constraints that are frequently manmade. Often the water is imagined in swimming pools, fishtanks, garden ponds, baths or even glasses, suggesting that the person's energies are limited by artificially created restrictions.

People often feel frustrated or angry that they are held back by such constraints. Marjorie imagined her dissolved tensions taking the form of a swimming pool full of people, and realized that most of her energy went into supporting others.

Mark, who imagined a powerful river cutting a downward V-shape into solid rock, realized that this was taking all his energy but was achieving nothing, since it was not going forward but to a dead end. He recognized that the "depression" the water was creating in the rock corresponded with his psychological state.

Others see the water as bursting its banks, "welling up" or widening its existing boundaries, while others are alarmed to find that it is shrinking or seeping away.

To understand the significance of these images it is important to remember that the water is the product of tensions dissolving in the mind and body. By relating its features back to the source of tension in the head or body, you may be able to identify the source of your tension.

6

ENERGY BALANCING THROUGH COLOR

The previous exercise may have helped you to gain insight into your tensions and the kinds of energy you tend to block, where these blockages are in your body, and how they arise. The exercise should also provide a way of dissolving these blockages, enabling your energies to flow more freely.

The following exercise will give you insight into the way your energies are being used at any time, and offer a way of balancing them so as to attain and maintain optimum health.

EXERCISE 3

Imagine you are sitting directly under a warm sun that is progressively soothing aches, pains and tensions from your mind and body. It seems that the rays of light streaming from the sun are flooding you with protective warmth. You are sitting under a waterfall of light, and you allow yourself time to experience this as fully as possible, to relax and feel at ease.

Imagine that the light cascading from above enters the pores of skin on the crown of your head, where there is a wheel which distributes the light throughout your head. As you observe this, note its size, the direction and character of its movement and how well it is distributing light. Pay careful attention to the predominant color of light being distributed. As you are doing so, notice that the wheel is like a pinwheel, distributing sparks of light that shower outward and downward. As you follow these downward, you see that there is another wheel situated at a point midway between your eyebrows, and that it too is distributing light. Once again, note all the features of this wheel, noting its size, direction and speed of movement and its predominant color.

As you follow the sparks it sends downward, you realize there are five more wheels positioned along the length of your body at points corresponding with the center of your throat, the middle of your chest, above and below your navel, and at the base of your spine. In turn you look at each of these wheels as they distribute light, noting in each case their size, direction and character of movement, and predominant color.

Having observed each wheel closely, look at the entire array of wheels. Note whether they are aligned, and how they compare with each other. Are they similar in size, lying in the same plane, moving in the same direction and at the same speed, or do they differ? If so, note how. Do they appear coordinated so that the light flows easily between them?

Now look at the base of your spine. Light is seeping from it. You appear to be sitting at the center of a growing pool of light that is extending away from you in a series of concentric circles. Notice the colors of each of these bands of light, and whether they are pale, dark, dense or patchy. Try to see where in your body any dark blotches or patches of color are coming from. Imagine this pool of light spreading out and joining with pools of light being produced by other people and things, first those nearest to you, then those farther and farther away. You now see yourself, all people and all things floating in an endless sea, each like a small ripple or wave on its vast surface. Be aware that all things are interconnected and that you affect everything by your thoughts, feelings and actions, just as you are affected by their thoughts, feelings and actions.

Now return your attention to the wheels of light in your body. Try and regulate them so that the flow of light from one to the other is smooth and harmonious; the sparks they emit are distributed through and around your body as a rainbow of color, and the pool of light in which you are sitting is pale, translucent and iridescent, like mother of pearl.

Having done so allow the image to fade, gradually returning yourself to normal, and record your experience.

COMMENTARY

This exercise provides a way of conceptualizing the structure of the chakra–aura system. Since imagery provides reliable information about subtle energies, the exercise gives you a way of assessing your energy at any time. Because imagery can also influence these subtle energies, you can also redirect and balance them.

I provide no introduction to this exercise to avoid creating expectations. Most people who undertake it have no prior knowledge about chakras, the aura and the physical, psychological and spiritual characteristics traditionally attributed to them. All the same, the correspondence between them is consistently striking, and usually enough to persuade the most skeptical of their validity.

Various features of the wheels as imagined are significant. People generally have little difficulty in visualizing the energy wheels of the body, although they may find that some are missing or difficult to picture in detail. Some people imagine that one or more wheels are missing. Women particularly report that the throat wheel is missing completely, or is erratic or sluggish in its movement, which may indicate that many find it difficult to express themselves.

More usually, all the wheels are imagined, but some are not working properly. Sometimes they appear wobbly, "on pins" like pinwheels, and erratic or eccentric in movement, suggesting that these energies are not easily expressed. Anxiety may be a contributory factor, as the phrase "being on pins" suggests. Lynn, for example, described her throat wheel as "bumpy" in movement, as though it wanted to move freely but couldn't.

In many cases the wheels differ in size and speed, with each one becoming progressively larger and slower. This conforms to traditional wisdom, which holds that the vibrations of each chakra become progressively more dense, heavy and lower in frequency down the length of the spine. Often all the wheels are of the same size. Generally, the size of a wheel is an indication of its robustness and energetic potential. Small wheels suggest limited energy, whereas large ones suggest the opposite.

The size of the wheel and the quality of its movement are interrelated. A sluggishly moving small wheel may suggest that the limited energy available is being conserved, whereas rapidly moving small wheels may be susceptible to burnout. Slow-moving, large wheels may be inefficient energy transmitters and large, fast-moving wheels may be chaotic and affect the functioning of the other wheels. However, in many cases there is no gradual progression in size or velocity of the wheels, but a chaotic mixture of large and small wheels moving at different speeds and without uniformity.

Most commonly some wheels are imagined moving very slowly, sluggishly or not at all, or very rapidly. Wheels that move quickly suggest overactivity. Overactivity in the wheel just above the navel is often described. This is the third or solar plexus chakra, which is associated with the color yellow and "heady" intellectual concerns and forcefulness. Where overactivity occurs this invariably indicates stress, resulting from the mind always being "on the go." This can increase the susceptibility to stress-related diseases. Where the heart or fourth wheel is overactive the emotions are likely to be overworked and drained, which can affect immunity to physical and emotional disorders.

Where the lower two wheels are overactive "sparks might fly," quite literally, because these relate to strong passions. Where the red wheel is overactive these passions may become overheated, leading to excess anger or aggression, violence and sexual deviance. Overactivity in the second wheel (navel chakra) may produce hyperactivity, which if unchecked may lead to physical exhaustion, excessive eating or drinking and digestive disorders.

Overactivity in the throat or fifth wheel may be associated with talking too much, a tendency to gossip, superficiality, throat problems and even hyperthyroidism. Underactivity reflects the opposite tendencies. Sluggishness in the throat wheel is likely to be associated with hesitancy in speech and self-expression and — in extreme cases — with hypothyroidism or an underactive thyroid.

Sluggishness in the heart wheel is likely to be associated with dulled emotional responses, indifference and reduced immunity. In the yellow wheel (solar plexus chakra) it may reflect intellectual dullness or lack of development, and feelings of powerlessness. Underactivity in the second wheel is associated with lack of drive and stamina and poor digestion; and lack of physical vitality, sex drive and productivity with the red wheel.

The direction and quality of movement usually varies considerably from wheel to wheel. Some wheels lie and move in a different plane to others, which can cause problems if the flow of energy from one wheel to another is disrupted. Wheels moving on a horizontal plane tend to distribute light only downward, rather than in all directions, and may be considered less efficient than wheels moving in a vertical plane. In some cases all the wheels move harmoniously in the same direction.

More typically, one or more wheels move counterclockwise. These effectively push out the energy available to them rather than distributing it within the body, thereby blocking this potential. The energy then manifests in the aura of the individual as color, and in the present exercise as color in the pool of light surrounding the person.

The colors of the wheels are always a good indicator of their functioning. It is highly variable, not only from person to person but over time. Many people describe the wheel colors in a way that is fully consistent with the rainbow sequence colors traditionally assigned to the chakras. Where the wheels vibrate harmoniously, a pure bright light may be observed. Others imagine each wheel emitting white light, which is a composite of all color. Some imagine rainbow colors emanating from each wheel. This imagery suggests a state of balance. But if certain wheels appear to be erratic, over or underactive or moving counterclockwise, this suggests that the current healthy situation is unlikely to continue. Clear "fluid" light emissions are also associated with wheels that are working well, and gold and silver emissions appear to indicate a harmoniously balanced system.

In many cases the colors traditionally associated with the chakras have been displaced. Thus someone may imagine yellow predominating in some or all wheels, indicating the predominance of mental energy and a tendency to rationalize everything. Where red appears in wheels other than the base it indicates anger and aggression. When it appears in the second wheel it suggests overexcitement, hyperactivity, heated passions and potential stomach problems. When it appears at the solar plexus the person may have angry thoughts and appear dominant, rude and threatening to others.

In the heart wheel, red represents "fire" in the heart, and thus passionate love. If the red deepens into black this may suggest thwarted passion and a "broken" or "bleeding" heart. Red in the throat wheel indicates frequent inflammation in that area and a tendency to express irritation. Jenny, who imagined red sparks being emitted by this otherwise blue wheel, admitted that she frequently tends to "spark off" rows and ill feeling by her angry outbursts. Where red appears in the brow wheel it may be a sign of mental illness, and it may indicate intense spirituality when it appears at the crown.

Orange is the color of activity and it rarely occurs other than in the lower wheels. In the base wheel it suggests an active sex life, and in the solar plexus wheel, a lively mind. Yellow, the color of rationality, often displaces other colors and indicates the tendency to analyze everything. When it appears in the base wheel it suggests that sex tends to be governed by the mind, and in the second wheel it suggests that gut feelings and passions are under rational control. Where it occurs in the heart wheel it indicates that the head rules the heart. Yellow appearing in the throat wheel is often a sign of the need to be seen to be clever. Some yellow in the brow wheel indicates insightful understanding, whereas too much can suggest skepticism. When it appears in the purple wheel, yellow shows that spiritual issues are dealt with intellectually rather than known and experienced directly.

Many people lack green in the heart wheel, showing that their heart isn't in their current endeavors. Dark green in this wheel indicates possessiveness and envy, as the well-known phrase suggests. When it appears in the second wheel it suggests emotional sensitivity, but if excessive it may indicate emotional vulnerability and sensitive digestion. In the red wheel it indicates that the heart is in one's sex life. If green does not appear in the solar plexus wheel this indicates a detached and analytical approach to life. Similarly, some green in the throat wheel is desirable, otherwise the person communicates little warmth and kindness and lacks sincerity. Turquoise, which combines blue and green, is associated with sincerity and genuineness, and often appears in this wheel. Too much green in this wheel, however, indicates too much kindness and the possibility of being exploited. Green in the brow wheel indicates generosity of spirit and in the crown wheel, compassion.

Wherever it appears, sky blue is suggestive of coolness. In the base wheel it indicates a cool attitude toward sex, and in the second wheel it is a sign of poor health and appetite. In the solar plexus it indicates a cool, clear head, whereas in the heart wheel it indicates emotional detachment and difficulty in forming relationships. When blue appears in the brow wheel and in the crown it indicates healing ability. Dark blue, or indigo, indicates impartiality wherever it appears, and purple or violet reflects aesthetic and spiritual qualities.

Generally the colors seen in the pool of light around the base wheel tend to correspond with anomalies in the relevant wheels. As such, the imagery reflects the correspondence between chakra functioning and the appearance of the aura.

People who describe their base wheel as black may feel that they have no vitality whatsoever. Brown indicates stagnant energies and withdrawal. In the base wheel it indicates lack of sexual fulfillment, and in the second wheel a lack of physical and emotional vitality. In the solar plexus it may be a sign of mental withdrawal and depression.

In the heart wheel brown is often a sign of grief, loss and susceptibility to disease. Brown in the throat wheel indicates a tendency to withdraw from communication with others and to speech problems. In the brow, brown indicates a tendency to withdraw from the outside world, and in the crown wheel it is connected with loss of faith, belief and purpose in life.

Many traditional practices are based on the belief that it is possible to receive information about subtle energies by way of imagery, and so chakra functioning can be reliably and accurately assessed in this and other ways. These practices also advocate visualization as a way to influence mental and bodily functions. Modifications of imagery such as speeding or slowing certain wheels, changing the direction or quality of movement, effecting repairs in damaged or dysfunctional wheels, and changing their color, may have benefits. This is the experience of many people who have described changes in their mental and physical condition corresponding with deliberately induced changes in their imagery.

The first time Sally tried this exercise she discovered that all her wheels were uncoordinated and moving sluggishly. She repeated the exercise daily for some time, imagining that the wheels were moving harmoniously and fairly forcefully in the same direction until she could "see" that they were emitting white light. As she did so, Sally noted considerable improvements in her overall health and well-being, both psychological and physical. Andrew noted a change in the direction of his brow wheel over a three-month period, and attributed this to the increased insight he had gained as a result of using imagery in the development of self-awareness.

PART THREE

——

DEVELOPING
YOUR TRUE COLORS

7

BREATHING IN COLOR

The exercises in Part Two may have given you some insight into the colors with which you resonate and those with which you don't; the personal energies these relate to; the extent to which you are using your energies effectively; the energies that you tend to block, and their implications for your life and general well-being.

The following exercises will help you to "own" the energies you currently disown, reject or project on to others and the environment, and to experiment by bringing more color into your life. This should enable you to promote all your energies and express your full potential.

Most people respond to unpleasant experiences by blocking their feelings. To do this they have to stop or slow down the energy flow through the relevant chakra, which affects its functioning in several ways. It may become blocked with stagnant energy, spin irregularly or counterclockwise, become disfigured or distorted, and eventually result in the development of a physical problem. This process not only generates illness but also the individual's reality, as Barbara Ann Brennan explains:

> Since chakras are not only metabolizers of energy, but also devices that sense energy, they serve to tell us about the world around us. If we "close" chakras, we do not let information come in. *Thus, when we make our chakras flow counterclockwise, we send our energies out into the world, sense what the energy is that we send out and say that this is the world. This is called projection in psychology.* (Italics in the original text.)

Thus energy that should be drawn into the chakra is projected out into the energy field surrounding the body, where it manifests as color, forming the filters through which the person sees the world. It colors his or her outlook on life, and determines the way he or she seems to others. The person who closes the base chakra energies relating to basic energies and functions will project the corresponding energy into his environment and will tend to "see red." His anger and aggression will tend to be projected on to others and, because he believes these energies arise in them rather than himself and are directed to rather than by him, he will probably feel insecure and lacking in confidence, act defensively and feel justified in doing so. He will seem angry, irritable and somewhat unstable to others.

The person who closes off his gut feelings will have passionate views, and will seem excitable, easily aroused and difficult to others. People who close their solar plexus energies will project their mental powers, power and mastery on to others. Accordingly they will see others as intimidating and powerful and themselves as victims. To others they will appear passive and even cowardly (or "yellow"). Everything will be colored by emotion for those who project their heart energy. They will see others as more valued and accepted than themselves, and will appear envious and re-sentful, as in the phrase "green with envy." They may have difficulty forming and maintaining relationships.

The person who projects his throat energies may see others as cool and distant and be seen by them as remote, reserved and uncommunicative, or shy. Someone who projects brow energies will see "as through a glass darkly." Everything will appear to be mystifying, impenetrable and unclear to him, and to others he will appear subdued, depressed, "blue." When someone projects crown energies, she will tend to see life through a purple haze and will have difficul-ty perceiving ordinary reality. To others she will seem "way out," detached and unworldly.

Closure of any chakra represents complete denial of feeling in a certain area. It is clearly an extreme reaction which, if sustained, will inevitably have unfortunate psychological and physical consequences. More typically, chakras are not completely closed but partially blocked so that some but not all of their energy is projected outward. This will color the person's outlook, but less consistently than if the chakra is completely closed. The first step in healing with color is to reverse the tendency of people to project certain energies and thereby "color" their life in ways that might lead to problems. From the exercises in Part Two, particularly Exercise 3 (page 76), which relates to chakra functioning and the appearance of the aura, you may have a fairly good idea of the energies you typically project outward and the ways these "color" your outlook on life and influence your well-being.

One way in which you can reverse this process is by breath-ing in color. This has long been a feature of traditional heal-ing practices and is widely used in contemporary color therapy. There are numerous variations of this practice, and it is advisable to experiment with several until you find one that seems best suited to your needs.

EXERCISE 4

The basic technique involves simply sitting or lying and establishing an easy, rhythmic breathing pattern. Then, as you focus on your breathing, imagine breathing in color. If you realize that you tend to block certain energies, focus on the relevant chakra and imagine breathing light of an appropriate color into it. Try not to think of this color, because thought is itself a "yellow" energy, but to sense it as fully as possible. If you are uncertain which energies you tend to block, just focus on your breathing and receive any color that emerges. As it does so, continue to breathe in the color and note any sensations that arise.

If you find that breathing in color is difficult — this usually happens if you are trying too hard — simply allow yourself to relax by breathing in sunlight. Imagine that you are sitting or lying in warm sunshine and breathing its energy into your body. Be aware of any thoughts, impressions, sensations or other experiences that arise as you do so.

COMMENTARY

Many people find that it is very easy to imagine breathing in sunlight and much less easy to imagine breathing in color. Some find it helpful to breathe in through their nose and out through their mouth, and in the Chinese tradition, to imagine that as they breathe in light it travels down their spine to its base and then upward, filling the body with light and pushing out "fog" through the mouth. Breathing in this way for a few minutes is usually enough to promote relaxation. When this happens you may find that colors begin to present themselves quite spontaneously. If they do, just carry on breathing in that way, being aware as you do so of any sensations or impressions.

A fascinating account of the insights and benefits that can derive from color breathing is provided by Jane. She first tried to breathe in the color she thought appropriate to her most obvious energy blocks as revealed in previous exercises and found it very difficult. So she imagined simply sitting under a warm sun and focusing her attention on her crown chakra. Suddenly and unexpectedly she gained a startling insight into how she was blocking her energy. She realized that the religious indoctrination of her childhood had "turned her off" religion. Her convent school education had left her with various hang ups and led to her rejecting the principles and practices of organized religion.

Jane realized that much of her denial of religion resulted from being hurt by one particularly punitive teacher, and that her experience had colored her attitude to the religious in general. As she did so she "saw" a vivid purple and by breathing in harmony with it she felt a great sense of relief. She discovered blockages in her throat chakra in relation to the way she expressed herself in certain contexts. Since she had always thought of herself as very self-expressive, this surprised her, but again Jane realized that painful experiences — this time in the workplace — had led her to suppress a good deal there. She found that as this insight emerged, so too did a vivid color, in this case a brilliant sky blue.

By now totally absorbed in the process, Jane continued to examine each chakra in turn, and found that in each case she tended to block the energies in ways she had not appreciated before, and that fear of being hurt had led to this restriction of her energies. Subsequently she found that simply by focusing on each chakra, the appropriate color would emerge and she could further her insights into its functioning. Over time Jane found significant changes occurring as she did so, along with greatly enhanced feelings of well-being.

8

LETTING COLOR
GO TO YOUR HEAD

Pat has participated in several of my workshops and also in one-to-one therapy with me. In one session she revealed that when she had attempted the wheel exercise (see Chapter Six) she had unaccountably found herself imagining hats. The experience had been so powerful that she had not only written it down but had also drawn some of the images she had received and brought them along to show me. When exploring these pictures with her and the valuable insights she got from them, I realized she had hit on a potentially useful exercise. I developed it systematically and "tested" it on other people.

Some time later, Pat told me of her surprise and delight to find a book in her local library by the psychologist Edward de Bono. She had been attracted by its title *Six Thinking Hats*. She was even more astonished on reading it to discover the striking similarity between her spontaneous imagery and that in the book. In his book, de Bono advocates wearing six different hats in order to promote different styles of thinking:

A *white hat* for neutral, objective, factual thinking.

A *red hat* for thinking that allows feelings, emotions, hunches and intuition of the thinker or others to be explored.

A *black hat* for thinking that is specifically concerned with negative assessment — pointing out what is wrong, or in error, and identifying risks, dangers and disadvantages.

A *yellow hat* for positive, constructive and optimistic thinking that explores and finds logical support for value and benefit, producing concrete proposals and suggestions, and "making things happen."

A *green hat* for creative thinking that is adaptable and generates new concepts and perceptions.

A *blue hat* for controlled, organized, disciplined thinking of the kind expected in summaries, overviews and conclusions.

The basic message of de Bono seems to be: "If the cap fits, wear it." A similar principle applies to the following exercise.

EXERCISE 5

Sitting or lying comfortably with your eyes closed, focus your attention on your pubic bone. Allow yourself some time to become aware of the sensations in this area. As you do so, allow the image of a red hat to form as vividly as possible and note your reactions to it. Try it on your head and wear it. Observe where you go and what you do while you have it on, and your feelings and thoughts as you do so.

Now focus your attention on the area some two inches below your navel, becoming aware of the sensation there. As you do so, allow the image of an orange hat to form. Put it on and wear it, observing where you go, what you do, how you feel and think.

In the same way, imagine a yellow hat forming in response to the sensations you experience just above your navel in the solar plexus; a green hat forming at the center of your chest; a sky blue hat at your throat; a dark blue hat in the center of the eyebrows; and a purple hat at the crown of your head. Imagine trying on and wearing each hat, noting your behavior, feelings and thoughts as you do so.

When you have allowed all the images to form, open your eyes and record what happened.

COMMENTARY

Most people thoroughly enjoy this exercise and are amused by it. Red energy relates to the base chakra, which is associated with basic vitality, sexuality and productivity. It energizes the feet, legs and pelvis and its function is to maintain a basic sense of grounding or security. People with positive red energy are likely to have their feet firmly on the ground, to feel rooted and have a good sense of reality.

In response to this exercise people frequently imagine themselves wearing red hats when engaged in physical activities, especially when participating in or spectating at sporting events, and feeling lively, energetic, excited, flamboyant and sexy. "Red hat" activities are often associated with status, and therefore with a person's social "standing." Women in particular tend to feel confident, smart, sophisticated and "uplifted" in red. People tend also to feel more secure in their personal relationships when wearing red. By expressing more red energy in your life you may be able to enhance your energy, vitality, security and self-confidence.

Orange energy is associated with the second chakra, and with powerful instinctive feelings. It is basic, physical and unrefined. Orange hats reflect this, generally being associated with energetic activities such as sport, dance, play and laughter; and with childish interests such as parties, games, circuses and clowns — that is, all the activities most people feel obliged not to engage in as they grow up. Most adults fail fully to express their "orange" energies, and need to relax in this area.

This can be achieved by surrendering to the orange hat imagery rather than resisting it. When Bernard imagined himself in a large orange floppy hat in which he wanted to laugh hilariously at nothing at all until he fell over, he merely allowed himself a smile and a suppressed chuckle. He didn't want to be seen as a fool by others for laughing out loud. Few people fail to feel the benefit of a "belly laugh" and for this reason certain Indian traditions advocate a form of breathing that requires the person to rapidly and repeatedly expell their breath. This produces a "ha ha" sound, which when repeated quickly leads to genuine laughter and so is believed therapeutic. This can be combined with color breathing.

Green energy associated with the heart chakra relates to connectedness and relationship, not only with others but with all creation. Typically, when people imagine wearing green hats they reflect the outdoor life. "Robin Hood" styles are often described, as are waxed weatherproof hats, riding caps and fashionable styles. People wearing these hats may describe feeling "lovely" or engaged in an activity they love, whether this is dog walking or gardening. These feelings can be enhanced by expressing your green energy.

Sky blue energy is associated with the throat chakra, and thus with speech and self-expression. Those who imagine wearing hats of this color often describe feeling "cool"; this is typically reflected in boating or sailing hats and skiing caps. Wearing these hats can be a liberating experience, reflecting some activity a person has always wanted to try but never has, such as ice skating, dancing or skiing.

When wearing blue hats many people, especially men, express themselves in ways they often describe as silly, which is no doubt a reflection of the inhibiting effects of social pressure toward seriousness rather than frivolity. Indeed social convention precludes a good deal of male expression. John, who imagined himself wearing a blue nurse's cap and carrying a stethoscope, described himself as "helping people and doing silly things like that."

Women may also be liberated from stereotypes of appropriate feminine behavior when wearing blue hats. Cathy, who imagined herself in a blue mortar board at a graduation ceremony, recognized this as an indication that she fails to express her intellectual energies fully. Angela found that when wearing a blue hat she could be more assertive.

Dark blue is associated with the brow chakra, with insight, imagination and intuitive abilities. Commonly hats of this color are associated with occupational groups such as nurses, police and fire officers, train conductors, taxi drivers, chauffeurs, pilots, sailors and the armed services, which all share a commitment to serving others. This is intriguing because in ancient traditions the third eye or brow chakra is associated with service to God or gods, fellow human beings and other creatures.

Surprisingly, however, these commonplace hats do not often feature in the above exercise. The hats described tend to be idiosyncratic, such as a many-tiered Chinese pagoda. Sultan's hats are often described. They tend to reflect far-sightedness and heightened perception. Julie described herself in one such hat flying off on a magic carpet to "see what is going on elsewhere." Jamie saw himself wearing a turban with a huge central jewel that enabled him to see all kinds of distant and future happenings.

Purple is associated with the crown chakra, with spiritual energies, enlightenment and transcendence of ordinary reality. Archbishops' mitres, papal crowns, wimples, wizards' and witches caps, triangular or conical headwear such as those favored by pharaohs, have all been described in connection with this chakra. People typically describe feeling taller and "above things" when wearing these hats. Feelings of power, raised consciousness, otherworldliness, transcendence and ecstasy have also been reported, as well as a sense of purpose. These feelings can be enhanced through expressing purple energy.

By experimenting with the various hats in the exercise it is possible to experience the thoughts, feelings, actions and reactions that result from liberating the energies of your chakras rather than blocking them. So you will get some sense of how you might be if you were to encourage and develop the expression of your true colors rather than inhibit them.

9

MANAGING PAIN WITH COLOR IMAGERY

I have suggested that in order to avoid unpleasant feelings, people slow down or stop the transmission of energy from the relevant chakras, which eventually leads to psychological and physical problems. The experiences most likely to be avoided are those that cause pain, whether physical or emotional. Blocking pain in this way leads to tension, which often increases existing physical pain. It also sets up a chain of events that may produce disease — both psychological and physical — and further pain. Ultimately, being "at pains" to avoid pain by blocking unpleasant feelings is self-defeating. Indeed pain can be conceived as both a cause and effect of blocked energy.

As we have seen, color imagery provides a valuable indication of and insight into the nature and location of energy blockages within the body — not only of existing tensions and pain but also of potential pain. Imagery can also be used to relax these tensions and pain and to promote and regulate the healthy flow of energy within the body. It can be used to modify pain, and is valuable not only in assessing but also in managing and treating pain. The following exercise is both simple and highly effective.

EXERCISE 6

Relax as fully as possible in whatever way suits you best. Then identify areas of residual pain in your body, or those areas in which pain tends to occur. Focusing your attention on each of these areas one at a time, allow an image to form in response to the sensations you experience there. Try not to influence or censor it in any way. If nothing comes to mind, don't "try" to produce an image — simply allow yourself to relax further while keeping a steady focus. When an image arises note its features, paying particular attention to color, shape and size, and noting any thoughts, memories or impressions. Ask yourself what you can learn about your pain from this image. You may find that you can interact with it. If so, ask it what it is doing there and why; what it is doing or can do for you, and what you can do for it.

Now try to change the color of the image, and as you do so, notice any sensations in your body and your mental and emotional reactions. Then change its shape and its size. Experiment with as many changes as you can, and take note of your physical, mental and emotional reactions as you do so. Next, shrink the pain and project it out of your body as far as you can, until it is out of sight. If you wish to, allow the pain to reappear and to return to its former position in your body, noting as it does so any changes in sensation. Then allow the image to fade, return to ordinary awareness and record your experience.

COMMENTARY

When asked to draw their pain, adults and children usually use the colors black, red, orange, brown, and less often purple and green. The more intense the pain the more likely they are to use red and black and to produce large drawings. Children typically draw spiky, angular abstract shapes to depict acute pain, reflecting the sensation of "sharpness." Less acute pain is shown as smoother, with curved rather than jagged outlines. Adults are less likely to draw abstract shapes than children, and more likely to add words and phrases.

Few people have any trouble creating images of their pain. Close examination of the various features of the images can yield valuable insights. For many people, however, the effects of changing their imagery in various ways are striking and dramatic. By doing so they discover that they have a degree of control over their pain, and therefore their experience of it.

Some people find that changing the color of the pain has immediate effects. Changing red and orange pains to blue or green can produce relief. Tension and migraine headaches respond well to blue, which generally appears to have a soothing effect when substituted for other colors. Sensations that appear as "black and blue" respond well to red and orange; and when the color of pain is vivid, simply diluting it can bring about marked improvement in reducing the pain.

Experimenting with color should reveal which is most appropriate to a particular pain, but some indication as to the nature and source of the pain, and the most appropriate way of managing it, may be provided by the color or colors of the initial image. Whereas red and orange are associated with physical pains, the musculoskeletal system and the lower areas of the body, yellow pain suggests the possibility of rather more mental issues; mental stress should be considered as a major underlying or contributory factor, together with related things such as fear and anxiety.

Where green appears, emotional factors and personal relationships play a part. When blue is a factor you may need to consider who or what is a "pain in the neck" for you, or even whether you are a "pain" and how this affects your self-expression and the way you are seen by others. Dark blue also raises the possibility of mental or psychological factors such as depression underlying or contributing to pain. Purple pain may indicate despair and loss of hope, direction and purpose. Black, brown and grey all suggest negativity, with denial playing a significant role in the pain experience.

It may seem strange that the exercise allows people to restore their pain to its original site, and that instead people would be pleased to rid themselves of it and would not want it back. Yet for many people the idea of their pain disappearing completely produces anxiety. On closer examination it usually emerges that these people need their pain because it meets some important function in their life. It may be a way of gaining the attention of others; or it may relieve them from unpleasant and unwanted roles or obligations. If you find that you are one of those reluctant or unable to let your pain disappear entirely, ask yourself what function it serves in your life, and whether it is possible to meet this need in another, less painful way.

Changing the color, shape and size of pain can have immediate and lasting effects. You might expect that in most cases the relief experienced is only short-term and that the pain will return. Certainly if you expect the pain to return it probably will, because this amounts to inviting it to do so. However, if you can achieve even fleeting relief from pain this may be enough to persuade you that you have power to control it, and that with practice you can develop this ability and extend the pain-free periods.

During her first attempt at visualization of this kind, Cathy experienced relief from a long-standing hip injury resulting from years of dance training. This persuaded her to continue, and after two weeks she was pain-free and able to wear high-heeled shoes for the first time in years. June successfully treated a long-standing knee injury, and Fred overcame long-standing tennis elbow. Shirley gained significant relief from her rheumatoid arthritis by modifying her green imagery.

Many of those people who successfully use color imagery come to realize the truth of the words Kahlil Gibran relates in *The Prophet*:

> Much of your pain is self-chosen.
> It is the bitter potion by which the physician
> within you heals your sick self.

10

BRINGING COLOR INTO YOUR LIFE

———

Through imaginative use of color, it is possible to realize your full potential and therefore promote spiritual, psychological and physical well-being, or health in its true sense. These brief guidelines will help you to bring more color into your life.

Red energizes the feet, legs, pelvis, hip joints, base of the spine, prostate, testes and urogenital tract. It stimulates physical activity and vitality, feelings of security, stability, self-confidence and warmth.

To bring more *red* into your life:

- breathe in red
- visualize red
- meditate on the color red, red flowers, gemstones and crystals
- wear red
- surround yourself with red

- place in your surroundings and wear gemstones and crystals such as garnet, ruby, red jasper, bloodstone, black tourmaline and smoky quartz

- use essential oils myrrh, patchouli and vetivert in burners, inhalers, massage oils and baths

- eat red meat, red-skinned vegetables and fruit, such as beetroot, radishes, red peppers, tomatoes, cherries, strawberries, kidney beans, chili peppers, and spices such as clove, cumin, chili and cayenne pepper

Use it:

- in rooms or buildings where increased physical activity is required

- in children's playrooms

- if you feel tired, run down or physically weak

- if you are cold

- if you are starting a head cold

- if you have problems of physical mobility, pains or stiffness in your legs

- if you have sciatica

- if you suffer from lower back pain

- if you have varicose veins

- if you have poor circulation

- if you are anemic

- if you have reproductive problems

- if you are infertile

- if you are impotent

- if you have prostate problems

- if you feel alone, unsupported and insecure

Do not use:

- with hyperactive, violent or aggressive children and adults
- in work situations where potentially dangerous machinery is in use
- where concentration is needed, for reading
- in bedrooms
- if you are angry or feeling aggressive
- if you are bleeding or suffer from hemorrhoids
- if you have inflamed cuts and wounds
- if you have infectious wounds
- if you suffer from high blood pressure
- if you have heart problems
- if you have eyestrain
- if you are accident prone
- if you want to relax

Orange energizes the liver, spleen, pancreas, kidneys and bladder. It stimulates metabolism, digestion, detoxification, immunity to disease, physical and emotional energies, sexuality, athletic performance and physical appetites, and regulates the sugar and fluid balance of the body.

To bring more *orange* into your life:

- breathe in orange
- visualize orange
- meditate on the color orange, orange flowers, gemstones and minerals
- wear orange
- surround yourself with orange

- place in your surroundings and wear amber, carnelian, coral and peach aventurine

- use essential oils sandalwood, cardamom and ginger in burners, inhalers, massage oils and baths

- eat oranges, tangerines, mandarins, apricots, melon, persimmon, papaya, carrots, orange peppers, lentils, and spices such as cinnamon, cloves, ginger and ginseng

Use it:

- in playrooms, exercise rooms, dance studios and sports halls

- where social gatherings take place

- if you have low energy

- if you feel lethargic or bored

- if you want to increase vitality

- if you want to enhance your sexuality

- if you feel depressed

- if you are inhibited

- if you need more energy to cope with the demands of everyday activities

- if you want to feel happy

- if you want to be playful and have fun

- if you want to stimulate your appetite

- if you have bladder problems or urinary tract infections such as cystitis

- if you have rheumatism

- if you lack sex drive

- if you have feelings of sexual inadequacy

- if you don't experience orgasm

- if you have menstrual difficulties or female dysfunctions such as vaginal infections, ovarian cysts, endometriosis, fibroids

Do not use:

- in resting areas
- if you tend to overeat or drink
- if you overindulge in sexual or sporting activities
- if you suffer from any addictions
- if you use stimulants
- if you suffer from nausea
- if you tend to be argumentative, angry, irritable
- if you have intestinal problems, irritable bowel syndrome, colitis, pancreatitis, diabetes, liver and kidney problems, hepatitis, gallbladder problems or adrenal gland dysfunction
- if you suffer from incontinence
- if you want to relax

Yellow energizes the adrenal glands, the sympathetic nervous system and thereby the muscles, heartbeat, digestion and circulation. It stimulates the digestive tract, mental activity, mental clarity, verbal reasoning and will power.

To bring more *yellow* into your life:

- breathe in yellow
- visualize yellow
- meditate on the color yellow, yellow flowers and minerals
- wear yellow
- surround yourself with yellow

- place in your surroundings and wear citrine, topaz, tiger's eye, yellow zircon, yellow jasper, gold and gold topaz

- use essential oils citronella and lemon in burners, inhalers, massage oils and baths

- eat yellow peppers, corn, grapefruit, melons, bananas, lemons, pineapple, eggs, cheese, yellow lentils, chickpeas and spices such as turmeric, mace, mustard and saffron

Use it:

- in reading rooms and studies:

- where social gatherings take place and lively conversation is required

- in the decor of rooms and buildings in which children with learning difficulties work

- if you are suffering mental fatigue

- if you feel mentally dull

- if your decision making is poor

- if your memory is poor

- if you need to concentrate

- if you are taking an examination

- if you have difficulty learning anything

- if you need to be objective

- if you feel nervous or fearful

- if you feel disempowered and submissive

- if you want to feel optimistic and confident

- if you have poor digestion

Do not use:

- with hyperactive, behaviorally disordered or aggressive children and adults

- if you are feeling restless
- if you are suffering from stress or a stress-related disorder
- if you cannot switch off mentally
- if you want to rest and relax
- if you suffer from insomnia
- if you are aggressive or prone to violence
- if you suffer from stomach disorders
- if you suffer from stomach ulcers, acute indigestion or nausea

Green energizes the thymus gland. It stimulates the heart, lungs, bronchia, arms, hands, skin, secondary circulation and the immune system. It promotes positive feelings, compassion and sensitivity.

To bring more *green* into your life:

- breathe in green
- visualize green
- meditate on the color green, green plants, gemstones and minerals
- wear green
- surround yourself with it
- walk in the countryside, buy houseplants, take up gardening
- use essential oils pine, bergamot, inula and melissa in burners, inhalers, massage oils and baths
- place in your surroundings and wear emerald, malachite, tourmaline, green agate, beryl, green jade, green aventurine, chrysoprase and rose quartz
- wear copper
- eat all green fruits and vegetables, avocados, olives and mung beans

Use it:

- in any rooms, buildings, workshops or studios where peace and calmness is desired, sensitivity is needed or activities involve physical touch

- if you need to calm down

- if you are anxious

- if you feel bitter or resentful towards others or have relationship problems

- if you find it difficult to give of yourself to others

- if you lack compassion

- if you want to develop your sensitivity

- if you feel "out of touch"

- if you are working with your hands

- if your heart is not in any aspect of your life or work

- if you have hypertension

- if you have heart problems

- if you have circulation difficulties

- if you have breathing problems, asthma or bronchitis)

- if you suffer from immune deficiency

- if you have tumors, cancer or AIDS

- if you have arthritis or rheumatism

- if you suffer from allergies

- if you have skin disorders

- if you suffer from chronic disease

- if you have upper back and shoulder problems

Do not use:

- in laboratories or rooms where detached analytical thinking is required

• if you suffer from auto-immune disease.

Sky blue energizes the thyroid gland and thereby the metabolism, the body's temperature control. It stimulates the voice, self-expression, communication, personal responsibility and hearing.

To bring more *blue* into your life:

• breathe in blue

• visualize blue

• meditate on blue, the sky, sea, water, the color blue, blue flowers, gemstones and minerals

• wear blue

• surround yourself with blue

• place in your surroundings and wear turquoise, chrysocolla, blue topaz, sodalite, aquamarine, azurite and kyanite gemstones and minerals

• use essential oils lavender, chamomile and geranium in burners, inhalers, massage oils and baths

• eat fish, blue-skinned fruits such as plums and blueberries, and asparagus

Use it:

• in bedrooms, resting areas, clinics, any room or building used for clinical procedures, dairies, cold stores

• if you need to calm your mind or nerves

• if you want to relax

• if you want to cool down physically, mentally or emotionally

• in cases of fever

• if you suffer from insomnia

• in cases of shock

- if you are bleeding
- if you have boils, hemorrhoids, inflamed or septic cuts and wounds, burns or sunburn
- if you have swollen glands
- if you suffer from psoriasis, skin conditions or irritations
- if you have insect bites or stings
- if you have ear, nose or throat problems
- if your voice is weak or you lose your voice
- if you cannot speak up for yourself
- if you suffer from embarrassment
- if you have a speech impediment
- if you have a stiff neck
- if you suffer from headache, tension headaches or migraine

Do not use:

- if you feel cold and shivery
- if you suffer from thyroid deficiency or slow metabolism

Dark blue or **indigo** energizes the pineal gland. It stimulates the lower brain, the central nervous system and the endocrine system — notably the hormones serotonin and melatonin. It thereby stimulates hormonal activity throughout the body, unconscious processes, imagination, insight, intuition and psychic abilities.

To bring more *indigo* into your life:

- breathe indigo
- visualize indigo

- meditate on indigo and dark blue, the late evening sky, blue minerals and gemstones

- wear indigo

- surround yourself with indigo

- place in your surroundings and wear gems and minerals such as lapis lazuli, sodalite, sapphire and azurite

- use essential oils patchouli and frankincense in burners, inhalers, massage oils and baths

- eat dark blue vegetables and fruits such as eggplants, plums, blueberries and grapes

Use it:

- in rooms where contemplation and meditation take place

- if you need to calm your nerves

- if you are agitated

- if you have problems sleeping

- if you feel restless

- if you need to think clearly and with insight

- if you lack imagination

- if you need to use or develop your intuition

- if you suffer from migraines

Do not use:

- in play rooms or centers of physical activity

- if you are depressed

- if you suffer from Seasonal Affective Disorder (SAD), eating disorders such as anorexia and bulimia nervosa, infertility or menstrual irregularities

- if you suffer from mental illness

- if you have nightmares

- if you feel melancholy and sad
- if you fear paranormal or psychic phenomena
- if you are taking sedatives

Purple or **violet** energizes the pituitary gland. It stimulates the upper brain and the nervous system, and creativity, inspiration, aestheticism, artistic ability and high ideals.

To bring more *purple* into your life:

- breathe purple or violet
- visualize purple or violet
- meditate on the color purple, purple flowers, mountains, gemstones and minerals
- wear purple and violet
- surround yourself with purple or violet
- walk in the mountains
- place in your surroundings and wear amethyst, alexandrite, sugalite, purple fluorite, selenite, diamond, clear quartz and aragonite
- use essential oils lavender, elemi and frankincense in burners, inhalers, massage oils and baths
- eat purple-skinned fruits and vegetables such as eggplants, grapes, asparagus and red cabbage

Use it:

- where you want to inspire artistic, creative, aesthetic and imaginative activities and spirituality, facilitate clear focus and awareness and meditation
- in theaters, children's classrooms
- if you need inspiration
- if you lack imagination
- if you need clarity of mind and purpose

- if you wish to meditate
- if you want to engage in visualization
- if you want to develop spiritually
- if you lack faith in yourself, others or the divine
- if you have lost your faith
- if you are striving for meaning and purpose in life
- if you are depressed
- if you suffer from paralysis or debilitating conditions such as multiple sclerosis

Do not use:

- in rooms used for entertaining or where you want to encourage conversation
- in rooms and buildings occupied by the mentally ill, especially those suffering delusions or depersonalization or with a tendency to be withdrawn
- if you have serious psychological problems
- if you have problems with alcohol or drugs
- if you feel alienated

HELPFUL ADDRESSES

The International Association of Colour Therapy
(affiliated with the Institute of
Complementary Medicine)
PO Box 3688
London SW13 0XA
England

International School for Colour Therapy
73 Elm Bank Gardens, Barnes
London SW13 0NX
England

Colour Energy Corporation
PO Box 1743, Station A
Vancouver V6C 2P7
British Columbia, Canada

Know Yourself Through Colour
Marie Louise Lacy
3a Bath Road, Worthing
Sussex BN11 3NU
England

The Maitreya School of Healing
33 Shaftesbury Road
London NI9 4QW
England

PRODUCTS

Color Energy Products
Nordraaksgt 8, 0260
Oslo, Norway

Hygeia Manufacturing Ltd
Hygeia Studios, Brook House
Avening, Tetbury, Glos GL8 8NS

RECOMMENDED READING

Aaranson, B.S., "Color perception and affect," *American Journal of Clinical Hypnosis* 14 (1971), 38–42.

Anderson, J., *Brain/Mind Bulletin* 15, 4 (1990), 1.

Bell, A.H. ed., *Practical Dowsing: A Symposium*, London: G. Bell & Sons 1965.

Birren, F., *Color Psychology and Color Therapy*, New York: Citadel Press, Carol Publishing Group 1992.

Brace, A., "Experts Hail Cure for Child Dyslexia," The *Mail on Sunday*, 27 June 1993, 10.

Branson, L., "Chromotherapy: Nature's Healing Rainbow," *Attitudes* (Spring 1988), 4–7.

Brennan, B.A., *Hands of Light: A Guide to Healing Through The Human Energy Field*, New York: Bantam 1988.

Costigan, K., "How Color Goes to Your Head," *Science Digest* (December 1984).

Davidson, J., *Subtle Energy*, Saffron Walden: C.W. Daniel Co. 1987.

Davis, P., *Subtle Aromatherapy*, Saffron Walden: C.W. Daniel Co. 1990.

De Bono, E., *Six Thinking Hats*, London: Penguin 1990.

Dougherty, T.J., "Photosensitization of Malignant Tumors" in S. Ecomon, ed., *Adjuncts to Cancer Therapy*, Philadelphia: Lea & Febinger 1980.

Dougherty, T.J., "Photoradiation Therapy — New Approaches," *Seminars in Surgical Oncology*, 6–16.

Gerard, R.M., "Differential Effects of Colored Lights on Psychophysiological Functions." Ph.D. thesis University of California at Los Angeles, 1958.

Gimbel, T., *The Book of Colour Healing*, London: Gaia Books Ltd 1994.

Gurudas, *Gem Elixirs and Vibrational Healing II*, California: San Rafael Press 1986.

Ivanov, A., "Soviet Experiments in Eyeless Vision," *International Journal of Parapsychology I* 1 (1965), 5–22.

Keenan, B., *An Evil Cradling*, London: Arrow 1993.

Krakov, S.V., "Color Vision and the Nervous System," *Journal of the Optical Society of America* (June 1942).

Lacey, J. R., "Neonatal Jaundice and Phototherapy," *Pediatric Clinics of N. America* 19 (4), (1972).

Legwold, G., "Color-boosted Energy: How Light Affects Muscle Action," *American Health* (May 1988).

Liberman, J., *Light: Medicine of the Future*, Santa Fe: Bear & Co. 1991.

Liberman, J., "Light, Medicine of the Future," *Caduceus* (Summer 1992), 22–5.

McDonald, S.F., "Effects of Visible Light Waves on Arthritis Pain: A Controlled Study," *International Journal of Biosocial Research* 3, 2 (1982), 49–54.

Motoyama, H. *Theories of the Chakras: Bridge to Higher Consciousness*, Wheaton, Illinois: Theosophical Society Publishing House 1988.

Novomeiskii, et al. reported in Ostrander, S. & Schroeder, L.S., *Psychic Discoveries Behind the Iron Curtain*, London: Sphere Books 1973.

Oren, D.A. & Brainard, G.C., "Treatment of Seasonal Affective Disorder with Green and Red Light," *American Journal of Psychiatry* 148 (4 April 1991).

Ott, J., "Color and Light: Their Effects on Plants, Animals and People," *Journal of Biosocial Research* 7, part 1 (1985).

Ott, J., *Health and Light: The Effects of Natural and Artificial Light on Man and Other Living Things*, Cold Greenwich, Conn: Devin-Adair Co. 1973.

Pellegrini, R.J., Schauss, A.G., Birk, T.J., "Leg Strength as a Function of Exposure to Visual Stimuli of Different Hues," *Bulletin of the Psychosomatic Society* 16, 2, 111–12.

Pierrakos, J.C., *Core Energetics*, Mendocino, California: Life Rhythm 1990.

Plack, J.J. & Schick, J., "The Effects of Color on Human Behaviour," *Journal of the Association for the Study of Perception* 9 (1974), 4–16.

Reich, W., *The Function of the Orgasm*, trans. Theodore P. Wolfe, New York: Oregon Institute Press, 1961.

Roney-Dougal, S.M., "The Psychophysiology of the Yogic-Chakra System," *Caduceus* (1989), 8–11.

Schauss, A.G., "The Physiological Effect of Color on the Suppression of Human Aggression: Research on Baker-Muller Pink," *International Journal of Biosocial Research*, 72 (1985), 55–64.

Schauss, A.G., "Tranquilizing Effect of Color Reduces Aggressive Behavior and Potential Violence," *The Journal of Orthomolecular Psychiatry* 8, 4 (1974), 218–21.

Schwarz, J. *Human Energy Systems*, New York: E.P. Dutton 1980.

Sun, H. & Sun, D., *Colour Your Life*, London: Piatkus 1992.

Vilenskaya, L., "Studies in Skin Vision," *applied Psi Newsletter* 1 (May/June 1982).

Wall, P.D., "The Gate-control Theory of Pain Mechanisms: A Re-examination and Restatement," *Brain*: 191, 1–18 (1989).

Watson, M., "Vital Force and Electricity," *Caduceus* (Autumn 1988), 24–6.

Westlake, A.T., *The Origins and History of Psionic Medicine*, London: Psionic Medical Society 1977.

White, R., "Rainbows of Health," *Caduceus* (Spring 1989).

Wills, P., *Colour Therapy: The Use of Colour for Health and Healing*, London: Element Books 1993.

Wohlfarth, H., "Experiments to Assert the Effects of Color-Stimuli Upon the Autonomic Nervous System," *Excerpta Medica Neurology and Psychiatry* 2 (1958).

INDEX

Exercises
  color breathing, 90–91
  energy balancing, 76–84
  energy blockages, 70–75
  hat exercise, 93–97
  pain management, 99–102
  relaxation, 60–68
Eyeglasses, tinted, 14
Eyeless sight, 14–15

Fifth chakra. *See* Throat chakra
First chakra. *See* Base chakra
Flower essences, 45
Fluorescent lights, 41
Foods
  and chakras, 20, 21
  and color healing, 42, 104,
    106, 108, 109, 111, 113, 114
Fourth chakra. *See* Heart chakra
Frequencies, energy, 52–53
Full-spectrum lamps, 16, 41
Full-spectrum light. *See*
  Sunlight; White (color/light)

Gem elixirs, 43, 44
Gemstones, 42–43
  and chakras, 20, 21
Gerard, Robert, 10–11
Gibran, Kahlil, 102
Gimbel, Theodore, 10, 13–14,
  39–40
Gold (color/light), and color
  exercises, 81
Greece, ancient, and healing
  with color, 5, 6
Green (color/light), 109–11
  and aura, 28
  and chakras, 20, 54–55
  clothing, 54
  and color exercises, 64, 66, 72,
    82–83, 93, 95, 100
  and essential oils, 43, 44, 109

foods, 109
  and growth experiments, 11
  and nervous system, 11
  and violence, 13
Grey (color/light)
  clothing, 54
  and color exercises, 72, 101
Growth experiments, 11

Halos, 17
Hara, 20, 23–24. *See also* Navel
  chakra
Hat exercise, 93–97
Healing with color. *See* Color
  healing
Health band (aura), 28
Heart band (aura), 28
Heart chakra, 20–21, 24–25, 26,
  28, 32, 35
  closing of, 88–89
  and color exercises, 80, 82, 83,
    95
  and essential oils, 43
Hermes Trismegistus, 5
History, of color healing, 3–16
Hormones, 15, 16, 22–23, 25
Human energy field, 18–37. *See*
  also Aura; Chakras
Humor theory (bodily fluids), 6
Hunt, Valerie, 31
Hygeia Studios, 10, 47
Hypertension, 10, 11

Imagery, 45–48, 84. *See also*
  Exercises
Indigo/dark blue (color/light),
  5, 112–14
  and aura, 28
  and chakras, 20, 25, 55
  clothing, 53, 54
  and color exercises, 83, 96,
    101

ULYSSES PRESS HEALTH BOOKS

DISCOVER HANDBOOKS

Easy to follow and authoritative, *Discover Handbooks* reveal an array of alternative therapies from around the world and demonstrate how to incorporate them into a program of good health.

Each book opens with information on the history and principles of the particular technique, then presents practical and straightforward guidance on ways in which it can be applied. Offering the tools needed to achieve and maintain an optimal state of health, the approach is one of personal improvement and self-reliance. Each of the books features: an introduction to the discipline; an explanation of its philosophy; step-by-step guide to its implementation; clear diagrams and charts; and case studies.

DISCOVER AYURVEDA
ISBN 1-56975-081-5, 128 pp, $8.95

DISCOVER COLOR THERAPY
ISBN 1-56975-093-9, 144 pp, $8.95

DISCOVER ESSENTIAL OILS
ISBN 1-56975-080-7, 128 pp, $8.95

DISCOVER FLOWER ESSENCES
ISBN 1-56975-099-8, 120 pp, $8.95

DISCOVER MEDITATION
ISBN 1-56975-113-7, 144 pp, $8.95

DISCOVER NUTRITIONAL THERAPY
ISBN 1-56975-135-8, 120 pp, $8.95

DISCOVER OSTEOPATHY
ISBN 1-56975-115-3, 132 pp, $8.95

DISCOVER REFLEXOLOGY
ISBN 1-56975-112-9, 132 pp, $8.95

DISCOVER SHIATSU
ISBN 1-56975-082-3, 128 pp, $8.95

A NATURAL APPROACH BOOKS

Written in a friendly, nontechnical style, *A Natural Approach* books address specific health issues and show you how to take an active part in your own treatment. Whether you suffer from panic attacks, endometriosis or depression, each book will provide you with a thorough understanding of your condition and detail organic solutions that offer immediate relief for your symptoms and effectively remedy their underlying causes.

Believing that disease is more than a combination of symptoms, these books offer integrated mind/body programs that take a positive, preventative approach. Since traditional drug therapy is not always the best solution (and can sometimes be the problem), these guides show how to use alternative treatments to supplement or replace conventional medicine.

ANXIETY & DEPRESSION
ISBN 1-56975-118-8, 144 pp, $9.95

ENDOMETRIOSIS
ISBN 1-56975-088-2, 120 pp, $8.95

FREE YOURSELF FROM TRANQUILIZERS
& SLEEPING PILLS
ISBN 1-56975-074-2, 192 pp, $9.95

IRRITABLE BLADDER & INCONTINENCE
ISBN 1-56975-089-0, 108 pp, $8.95

IRRITABLE BOWEL SYNDROME
ISBN 1-56975-030-0, 240 pp, $11.95

MIGRAINES
ISBN 1-56975-140-4, 156 pp, $8.95

PANIC ATTACKS
ISBN 1-56975-045-9, 148 pp, $8.95

THE NATURAL HEALER BOOKS

As home remedies and alternative treatments become increasingly accepted into the medical mainstream, people want information—not just hype and unproven claims—about the remedies they see in health food stores. *The Natural Healer* books detail how these natural remedies have been used throughout history and how to safely incorporate them into an overall plan for maintaining good health.

CIDER VINEGAR
ISBN 1-56975-141-2, 120 pp, $8.95

GARLIC
ISBN 1-56975-097-1, 120 pp, $8.95

THE ANCIENT AND
HEALING ARTS BOOKS

The Ancient and Healing Arts books recount the development of healing art forms that have been used for thousands of years. Beautifully illustrated with full color on every page, they discuss the benefits of these time-honored techniques and offer detailed instructions on their use.

THE ANCIENT AND HEALING ART OF
AROMATHERAPY
ISBN 1-56975-094-7, 96 pp, $14.95

THE ANCIENT AND HEALING ART OF
CHINESE HERBALISM
ISBN 1-56975-139-0, 96 pp, $14.95

OTHER HEALTH TITLES

THE BOOK OF KOMBUCHA
ISBN 1-56975-049-1, 160 pp, $11.95
Explains the benefits of and addresses concerns about Kombucha, the widely used Chinese "tea mushroom."

HEPATITIS C: A PERSONAL GUIDE TO GOOD HEALTH
ISBN 1-56975-091-2, 172 pp, $12.95
Identifies the causes and symptoms of hepatitis C and presents conventional and alternative treatments for coping with the disease.

KNOW YOUR BODY: THE ATLAS OF ANATOMY
ISBN 1-56975-021-1, 160 pp, $12.95
Presents a full-color guide to the structure of the human body.

MOOD FOODS
ISBN 1-56975-023-8, 192 pp, $9.95
Shows how the foods you eat influence your emotions and behavior.

YOUR NATURAL PREGNANCY: A GUIDE TO COMPLEMENTARY THERAPIES
ISBN 1-56975-059-9, 240 pp, $16.95
Details alternative therapies ranging from aromatherapy to yoga that can benefit pregnant women.

To order these books call 800-377-2542, fax 510-601-8307 or write to Ulysses Press, P.O. Box 3440, Berkeley, CA 94703-3440. All retail orders are shipped free of charge. California residents must include sales tax. Allow two to three weeks for delivery.

A lecturer in psychology at Keele University in England, Helen Graham has specialized in color research for a number of years and runs workshops on the use of color healing.